Transition to Nursing Practice: from student to registered nurse

Sara Miller McCune founded SAGE Publishing in 1965 to support the dissemination of usable knowledge and educate a global community. SAGE publishes more than 1000 journals and over 800 new books each year, spanning a wide range of subject areas. Our growing selection of library products includes archives, data, case studies and video. SAGE remains majority owned by our founder and after her lifetime will become owned by a charitable trust that secures the company's continued independence.

Los Angeles | London | New Delhi | Singapore | Washington DC | Melbourne

Transition to Nursing Practice: from student to registered nurse

Angela Darvill,
Melanie Stephens and
Jacqueline Leigh

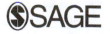

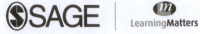

Learning Matters
An imprint of SAGE Publications Ltd
1 Oliver's Yard
55 City Road
London EC1Y 1SP

SAGE Publications Inc.
2455 Teller Road
Thousand Oaks, California 91320

SAGE Publications India Pvt Ltd
B 1/I 1 Mohan Cooperative Industrial Area
Mathura Road
New Delhi 110 044

SAGE Publications Asia-Pacific Pte Ltd
33 Pekin Street #02–01
Far East Square
Singapore 048763

Editor: Donna Goddard
Development editor: Eleanor Rivers
Senior project editor: Chris Marke
Project management: Swales & Willis Ltd,
Exeter, Devon
Marketing manager: Tamara Navaratnam
Cover design: Wendy Scott
Typeset by: C&M Digitals (P) Ltd, Chennai, India
Printed in the UK

Library of Congress Control Number: 2018939033

British Library Cataloguing in Publication data

A catalogue record for this book is available from the
British Library

ISBN 978-1-4739-7868-3 (pbk)
ISBN 978-1-4739-7867-6

At SAGE we take sustainability seriously. Most of our products are printed in the UK using responsibly sourced papers
and boards. When we print overseas we ensure sustainable papers are used as measured by the PREPS grading system.
We undertake an annual audit to monitor our sustainability.

Contents

TRANSFORMING
NURSING PRACTICE TNP

Transforming Nursing Practice is a series tailor-made for pre-registration student nurses. Each book in the series is:

- Affordable
- Mapped to the NMC Standards and Essential Skills Clusters
- Full of active learning features
- Focused on applying theory to practice

Each book addresses a core topic and has been carefully developed to be simple to use, quick to read and written in clear language.

> " An invaluable series of books that explicitly relates to the NMC standards. Each book covers a different topic that students need to explore in order to develop into a qualified nurse... I would recommend this series to all pre-registration nursing students whatever their field or year of study
>
> **Linda Robson**
> **Senior Lecturer, Edge Hill University**
>
> The set of books is an excellent resource for students. The series is small, easily portable and valuable. I use the whole set on a regular basis.
>
> **Fiona Davies**
> **Senior Nurse Lecturer, University of Derby**
>
> I recommend the SAGE/Learning Matters series to all my students as they are relevant and concise. Please keep up the good work.
>
> **Thomas Beary**
> **Senior Lecturer in Mental Health Nursing, University of Hertfordshire** "

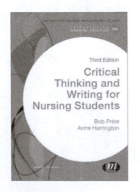

Third Edition
Critical Thinking and Writing for Nursing Students
Bob Price
Anne Harrington

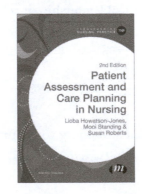

2nd Edition
Patient Assessment and Care Planning in Nursing
Lioba Howatson-Jones,
Mooi Standing &
Susan Roberts

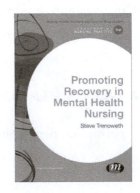

Promoting Recovery in Mental Health Nursing
Steve Trenoweth

You can find more information on each of these titles and our other learning resources at **www.sagepub.co.uk**. Many of these titles are also available in various e-book formats, please visit our website for more information.

Foreword

Transitions can be a very stressful time. You may be moving from one area where you were competent and confident and suddenly you are thrown into a new area where you don't know how everything works. Your competence and confidence can take a battering. Most of us don't like that feeling of uncertainty, of not knowing. We wonder whether we will be able to cope and learn all that is required of us. This can lead to a lot of doubts and worries and even feelings of being an imposter.

Our expectations of ourselves are usually quite unrealistic too. We expect that we should be fully competent in the new role from day one. To hit the ground running. Of course this is unrealistic but we still expect it.

The new environment and the support available also plays a huge role in transitions. If you are thrown in the deep end you may swim but you may also sink. That's why I was so pleased to be asked to write a foreword for this very valuable book. The content, the activities and self-reflection it encourages provide wonderful support for you as you make your transition from student to registered nurse.

Be brave and enjoy the transition.

Hugh Kearns

Lecturer and researcher at Flinders University, Adelaide, Australia

Director of Thinkwell

www.ithinkwell.com.au

About the authors

Angelina Chadwick is a lecturer in mental health nursing. She is a registered adult and mental health nurse with previous experience in both fields of practice. Angelina has held a variety of management and educational roles, leading to an MSc in leadership and management for health care practice. Research interests include leadership, professional development, physical health issues within mental health and the inclusion of high fidelity simulation in teaching.

Catherine Croughan is a Registered Nurse in the Adult field of practice and is a Lecturer in Adult pre-registration nursing and Programme Leader at the University of Salford. She has previous experience of cardiac and general nursing including roles in leadership and management and has a keen interest in education, particularly in relation to her research interests of professional practice and development. Catherine holds a higher degree in Health Studies alongside a Masters of Sciences in Nurse Education.

Dr Angela Darvill is a Senior Lecturer in Children and Young People's nursing at the University of Huddersfield. Angela has over 20 years experience in higher education and has been responsible for the education of nurses, mentors and lecturers. Angela's PhD was a study of newly registered children's nurses' transition into children's community nursing teams.

Chris Fisher is a lecturer in Adult Nursing at the University of Salford. His clinical background is acute medical nursing. Currently Chris teaches undergraduate nursing students. His research interests include widening participation in Adult Nursing.

Leyonie Higgins is a Children and Young People's lecturer at the University of Salford, teaching on undergraduate pre-registration and post qualifying nursing programmes. She was awarded a Senior Fellowship based on her collaborative work to integrate careers preparation and health and wellbeing into the pre-registration curriculum to ensure a successful transition from student to newly registered nurse.

Andrew Kay is a Careers Consultant at the University of Salford and has over 21 years' experience delivering careers support within higher education. In recent years he has worked closely with nursing and other health students to support and ensure a successful transition from student to professional.

Joanne Keeling is the manager of pre-registration nursing education at the University of Central Lancashire. She is a mental health nurse by background and has been working in higher education for over 15 years predominantly in pre-registration nursing programmes. Joanne's research interests lie in the areas of mental health promotion, with particular reference to the education and sporting environments, and the development of creative curricula. Joanne holds higher degrees in law and community and healthcare ethics and is currently studying for a PhD.

Dr Jacqueline Leigh is a Reader in Teaching and Learning Health Professional Education and is an Adult Nurse. She is an advocate for evidence based education, teaching and assessment and has significant experience in developing innovative curricula that meet workforce needs in health and social care. Jackie has set up and leads the Educational Research and Scholarship Cluster and is passionate about practice based learning and clinical leadership.

Denise Major is a retired lecturer in nursing, whose clinical expertise lies within neonatal nursing, in the sociological context of societal health and illness. Although no longer lecturing, Denise continues to promote the health and wellbeing of children and families through providing breast-feeding support for new-borns and their parents. Being interested in the complete student journey from recruitment to Registered Nurse, Denise's academic career focussed strongly on the quality of teaching and assessing in university and in clinical nursing practice. Her teaching and leadership spanned several modules, including the preparation of student nurses for their professional practice as newly registered nurses. Denise's higher degree research, and its follow-up study, provided an evidence base, from the students' perspective, of best practice learning-facilitation during their final year transition to the newly registered nurse role.

Iain Pearson has been a Wellbeing Advisor at the University of Salford since 2010. He works with students from a wide range of backgrounds offering emotional support for a wide range of issues such as anxiety, depression, stress, university transition and self-esteem. He provides one-to-one support and workshops, focussed on improving student wellbeing, and is a member of the University Mental Health Advisors Network.

Melanie Stephens is a Senior Lecturer in Adult Nursing and a health service researcher. She has led the School of Health and Society's Preparation for Role Transition Module for the past five years. Melanie is a health service researcher and a team member of the research programme for knowledge, health and place, with specific research interests in pressure redistributing properties of seating, tissue viability, and interprofessional working.

Tyler Warburton is a lecturer in Adult Nursing at the University of Salford with a clinical background in neonatal and theatre nursing. Having worked within a number of practice based education roles Tyler is passionate about the application of sound educational theory and principles within the clinical learning environment. He is currently pursuing research in the use of creative pedagogies within healthcare education.

Dr Mark Widdowson is a Senior Lecturer in counselling and psychotherapy at the University of Salford. He is a teaching and supervising transactional analyst and a UKCP registered psychotherapist. He is an active psychotherapy researcher and is the author of *Transactional Analysis: 100 Key Points and Techniques and Transactional Analysis for Depression: A Step-By-Step Treatment Manual*, published by Routledge in 2016. In addition to working in the university, he also has a small private practice in central Manchester working with individuals and couples.

Acknowledgements

The authors and publisher would like to thank the following for permission to reproduce copyright material:

John M. Fisher for permission to use the process of transition diagram (Figure 1.2).

McGraw Hill publishers for permission to use Borton's (1970, p89) 'reflective sequence' of 'What, So what, Now what'.

The authors and publisher would like to thank the following students for their feedback on the chapters of the book as they were in development.

Yasmin Ibison, BA Modern Languages, University of Birmingham

Niamh Jones, BSc Nursing Adult, University of Salford

Megan Kumeta, BSc Nursing Adult, University of Salford

Amy Lewis, BSc Nursing Children and Young People, University of Salford

Prudence S Mlambo, BSc Nursing Adult, University of Salford

Anna Muscolino, BSc Nursing Adult, University of Salford

Harriet Serwaa, BSc Nursing Mental Health, University of Salford

Maxine Womack, BSc Nursing Mental Health, University of Salford

Yasmin Lauren Woolf, BSc Nursing Children and Young People, University of Salford

Introduction

About this book

It is well recognised that entering the world of work is a stressful time for newly registered nurses. This is attributed to the perceived awareness of the stress of an increase in responsibility and accountability and perceived knowledge, skills and confidence deficits leading to feelings of stress and shock. Preparation for this transition can reduce these shock-like reactions and this book aims to guide students and newly registered nurses through this process.

Why transition to nursing practice: from student to registered nurse

This book helps student nurses and newly registered nurses navigate and overcome some of the common barriers to a smooth transition journey.

Book structure

This book has eight chapters and, in each chapter, applies 'real world' transition scenarios that help the reader apply theory to practice. The scenarios use gender neutral names. Gender neutral names are becoming increasingly accepted in the literature, in order to avoid stereotyping. Stereotyping in this way involves making assumptions about the characteristics of an individual that are based on a standard, simplistic characterisation of a person's gender and culture, in this case their name. According to the NMC Code (2015) nurses should avoid making assumptions and recognise diversity and individual choice. As authors, we are sensitive to the current legislation and policy in regard to this issue. However, individuals differ considerably and may adopt values and beliefs not congruent with the assumption we may have already made from their name. As healthcare practitioners we have to minimise assumptions in regard to issues such as sex, gender or culture when writing and delivering care.

Chapter 1 Managing the transition from student to registered nurse

This first chapter enables you to examine and analyse the concept of transition and consider the milestones and challenges you may face during the transition process. You will be able to undertake a variety of activities to consider the stages you may go through in your transition journey. This chapter will enable you to prepare for your transition and acquire strategies to develop transition resilience and take control of your learning and development to enhance your experiences of transition.

Chapter 2 Self-assessment of knowledge, skills and attitudinal values through critical reflection

Building upon your theoretical learning about transition in the first chapter, Chapter 2 lays the practical foundation of managing your own transition from student to registered nurse in an organised and timely manner, so that you gradually make your journey in planned, manageable steps. Utilising a variety of self-assessment tools, the chapter activities provide an opportunity to closely examine the knowledge, skills and attitudinal values that you have so far acquired during your time as a student nurse. By the end of the activities you should have identified your own personal, professional and academic learning needs that still require development, in order to meet NMC registration requirements. These learning needs can then be recorded and managed through a transition-focussed personal development plan, such as that explored in Chapter 3, to enable your smooth transition towards registration.

Chapter 3 Transition-focussed reflection and personal development planning

This chapter provides opportunity for critical thinking as a way to reflect deeply on all aspects of your professional development of knowledge, skills and attitudinal values, through the use of structured reflective models. With particular emphasis on your transition from student to newly registered nurse, the first part of the chapter provides a scenario and theoretical perspectives that will help you to further, assess and challenge your own professional development. This critical reflection can be used in conjunction with the self-assessment tools and SWOT/SNOB analysis introduced in Chapter 2. The latter half of Chapter 3 provides activities and worked examples to help you formulate your own, individualised, transition-focussed personal development plans (TFPDPs) from all of your reflective self-assessments.

Chapter 4 Looking after your health and wellbeing during role transition

This chapter focusses on how your personal health and wellbeing can be affected during role transition and in turn how this can influence how you behave and act professionally. It starts by reviewing definitions of health and wellbeing from nursing theory and progresses on to recognising when you might be physically and/or emotionally unwell with the opportunity to recognise signs and symptoms of ill health and negative habits. The chapter proceeds with exploring the impact of good and bad stress and recommends strategies to reduce stress and build resilience. Finally, the chapter offers support strategies that will aid in reducing or managing physical and emotional ill health.

Chapter 5 Learning theory for personal and professional development

This chapter explores the importance of understanding how you learn and how this knowledge can be used to support your transition from student to newly registered nurse. This chapter offers scenarios based around student nurses who are at different stages of their nursing programme and who demonstrate similarities and different preferences for learning. Completion of the learning activities will help you make sense of the range of learning theories and how they can be applied to your role transition. Theories include behaviourist, social learning, cognitive and social aspects of learning.

Chapter 6 Identifying and developing clinical leadership in relation to transition

This chapter explores the concepts of leadership and management using a scenario. Definitions of leadership and clinical leadership are provided. You will draw on concepts introduced in Chapter 2 such as the self-assessment SWOT analysis to enable you to develop individual transition focussed personal development plans. Development of your leadership skills will equip you to deliver high quality care that takes place within an ever-changing healthcare environment, ensuring the provision of high quality care for those within your service.

Chapter 7 Transition support

This chapter enables you to identify and comprehend the importance of transition support to help you develop into an autonomous practitioner. The chapter will focus on many topics from identifying support systems and the impact this can have on job performance, to the development of clinical decision making to and becoming an autonomous practitioner. You will be introduced to theories such as imposter syndrome and explore the change from mentorship to preceptorship or another form. This chapter also investigates the meaning of supernumerary status, the provision of feedback and other forms of support during your transition.

Chapter 8 Preparing for, developing and maintaining your nursing career

This chapter will enable you to enhance your understanding of the recruitment process and consider the evidence you will provide to meet your employers' expectations regarding your knowledge, skills and values to secure your first post. You will be able to review current job descriptions and personal specifications and consider collating your evidence to enable you to write your application form. Guidance will be provided on preparing for interview and finally suggestions for continuing professional development will be discussed. This chapter will enable you to consider planning and developing your learning and development needs for your continuing career.

Requirements for the NMC Standards for Pre-registration Nursing Education and the Essential Skills Clusters

The Nursing and Midwifery Council (NMC) has established standards of competence to be met by applicants to different parts of the register, and these are the standards it considers necessary for safe and effective practice. In addition to the competencies, the NMC has set out specific skills that nursing students must be able to perform at various points of an education programme. These are known as Essential Skills Clusters (ESCs). This book is structured so that it will help you to understand and meet the competencies and ESCs required for entry to the NMC register. The relevant competencies and ESCs are presented at the start of each chapter so that you can clearly see which ones the chapter addresses. There are *generic standards* that all nursing students irrespective of their field must achieve, and *field-specific standards* relating to each field of nursing; i.e. mental health, children's, learning disability and adult nursing. Most chapters have generic standards, and occasionally field-specific standards are listed.

This book includes the latest standards for 2010 onwards, taken from the *Standards for Pre-registration Nursing Education* (NMC, 2010).

Learning features

Learning from reading text is not always easy. Therefore, to provide variety and to assist with the development of independent learning skills and the application of theory to practice, this book contains activities, case studies, scenarios, further reading, useful websites and other materials to enable you to participate in your own learning. You will need to develop your own study skills and 'learn how to learn' to get the best from the material. The book cannot provide all the answers – but instead provides a framework for your learning.

The activities in the book will in particular help you to make sense of, and learn about, the material being presented. Some activities ask you to reflect on aspects of practice, or your experience of it, or the people or situations you encounter. *Reflection* is an essential skill in nursing, and it helps you to understand the world around you and often to identify how things might be improved. Other activities will help you develop key graduate skills such as your ability to *think critically* about a topic in order to challenge received wisdom, or your ability to research a topic and find appropriate information and evidence, and to be able to *make decisions* using that evidence in situations that are often difficult and time-pressured. Communication and working as part of a team are core to all nursing practice, and some activities will ask you to carry out team work activities or think about your *communication skills* to help develop these. Finally, as a registered nurse you will be expected to *lead and manage* your own team, case load or area of care, and so some activities focus on helping you build confidence in doing this.

All the activities require you to take a break from reading the text, think through the issues presented and carry out some independent study, possibly using the internet. Where appropriate, there are sample answers presented at the end of each chapter, and these will help you to understand more fully your own reflections and independent study. Remember, academic study will always require independent work; attending lectures will never be enough to be successful on your programme, and these activities will help to deepen your knowledge and understanding of the issues under scrutiny and give you practice at working on your own.

You might want to think about completing these activities as part of your personal development plan (PDP) or portfolio. After completing the activity write it up in your PDP or portfolio in a section devoted to that particular skill, then look back over time to see how far you are developing. You can also do more of the activities for a key skill that you have identified a weakness in, which will help build your skill and confidence in this area.

We hope that you enjoy this book and that through engaging with the range of activities offered this positively supports your smooth role transition.

Chapter 1

Managing the transition from student to registered nurse

Angela Darvill and Catherine Croughan

NMC Standards for Pre-registration Nursing Education

This chapter will address the following competencies:

Domain 1: Professional values

7. All nurses must be responsible and accountable for keeping their knowledge and skills up to date through continuing professional development. They must aim to improve their performance and enhance the safety and quality of care through evaluation, supervision and appraisal.
8. All nurses must practise independently, recognising the limits of their competence and knowledge. They must reflect on these limits and seek advice from, or refer to, other professionals where necessary.
9. All nurses must appreciate the value of evidence in practice, be able to understand and appraise research findings to their work, and identify areas for further investigation.

Essential Skills Clusters

This chapter will address the following ESCs:

Cluster: Care, compassion and communication

Entry to the register:

1. As partners in the care process, people can trust a newly registered nurse to provide collaborative care based on the highest standards, knowledge and competence.
8. Demonstrates clinical confidence through sound knowledge, skills and understanding relevant to field.
9. Is self-aware and self-confident, knows own limitations and is able to take appropriate action.

Cluster: Organisational aspects of care

16. People can trust the newly registered nurse to safely lead, co-ordinate and manage care.
1. Inspires confidence and provides clear direction to others.
2. Takes decisions and is able to answer for these decisions when required.
3. Bases decisions on evidence and uses experience to guide decision making.
5. Manages time effectively.

Chapter aims

After reading this chapter you will be able to:

- examine the concept of transition and analyse factors that may facilitate or inhibit the management of a successful transition from student to newly registered nurse;
- examine the theory and research evidence in relation to transition from student to newly registered nurse and its application to your transition;
- discuss the factors that may facilitate or inhibit your transition from student to newly registered nurse;
- assess the implications of transition theory for your transition.

Introduction

The chapter will begin by introducing a scenario of a newly registered nurse and a concept summary of transition from student to newly registered nurse. After this, we will explore the stages of transition to help you to understand the stages you might through in your transition journey and how to identify the process of your transition. There are activities for reflecting on your feelings and emotions during this process and identifying the challenges you may face and factors that can assist your transition journey. You might want to consider expanding your reading and knowledge base in this field by accessing the supporting material within this chapter.

Scenario

Gerry is a newly registered nurse entering a first post as a staff nurse and has chosen the clinical area from past placement experiences. Gerry is about to start this journey with a degree of excitement and is looking forward to a long and rewarding career in

(Continued)

(Continued)

nursing. The last three years have been about developing knowledge, skills and values and Gerry is now looking forward to moving on to the next stage.

However, Gerry has heard stories from other nurses about what the change was like for them and is approaching this change with feelings of trepidation and dread. Gerry has been reading the recent statistics from the NMC regarding nurses leaving the NMC register within the first three years of qualifying. However, Gerry is aware of the recent advances in support for newly registered nurses in order to retain the workforce.

During the last year Gerry has faced many challenges in preparing for transition and is now ready for this exciting challenge. Gerry has contacted the ward manager for guidance on induction and the new nurse induction programme that is in place in the employing organisation.

This chapter has started with the above scenario to help illustrate what transition is like for newly registered nurses. You may find yourself in a similar situation to Gerry and reflecting on your own and Gerry's experience will influence your perception and understanding of the process of transition and factors that can help for a smooth transition into the world of work. Understanding the concept and developing insights can help you to understand your own experience in the context of others' experiences. This chapter will provide you with baseline knowledge of transition as a starting point to the remaining chapters in the book. This will assist you in developing your transition skills.

Concept summary

What is transition?

Transition has been defined by Chick and Meleis (1986, p239) as the 'passage from one life phase, condition or status to another, embracing the elements of process, time span and perception'. This means your journey from student nurse to newly registered nurse is an alteration in your status, and involves your experiences and perceptions of the process itself. It not only involves changes and demands for you, but also how you respond to these. Transition from student to newly registered nurse is a temporary phase that involves a period of adjustment and change. Transition begins with the first anticipation of the change and it continues until stability occurs in the new status within a defined time frame. Everyone will experience this transition; however, you will interpret the experience from your own subjective and unique perspective.

The stages of transition

The period of transition is experienced in a series of stages. These stages are defined using the concept of 'Rites of Passage'.

> ## Concept summary
>
> Van Gennep (1960) coined the term rites of passage to describe various stages that he discerned as discrete over time, and named these rites of separation, rites of transition and rites of incorporation. According to van Gennep (1960) the first stage of any rites of passage is rites of separation. He asserted that this stage was characterised by the removal of the individual from their existing social position; and that they acknowledged that a prior way of life had ended. The next stage, an intermediate stage, was termed the rites of transition. This involved individuals appropriating the customs and rituals of the new social position that brought a sense of order. The rites of incorporation were characterised by the individual taking up their new status and identity, and then being accepted by the group (van Gennep, 1960).

Figure 1.1 depicts a summary of the stages and findings (Darvill, 2013) regarding the transition process.

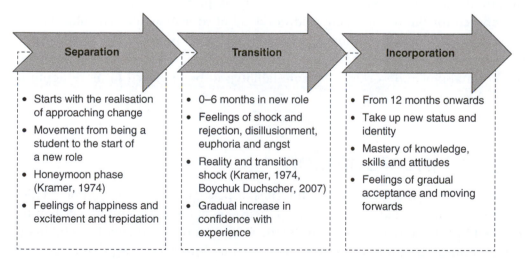

Figure 1.1   The stages of transition

Figure 1.1 is explained in more detail in the chapter.

Rites of separation

Within nursing, separation is characterised by your movement from being a student nurse to being a newly registered nurse. This movement is inevitable as you transfer from the comparative safety of a student to the unknown position of a newly registered nurse. This marks the end of your initial educational preparation and the beginning of your professional journey as a registered nurse.

As you approach the end of your undergraduate nurse education programme, like Gerry you may be experiencing feelings of excitement and trepidation. You may be looking forward to caring for patients independently and working autonomously. You may also be looking forward to your new professional status in your first job and the easing of financial stress. Like Gerry you may be considering choosing your first post in a clinical area where you have worked before. Your feelings about your first post may be affected by many things such as your past experiences and listening to what others say about the future work place.

Rites of transition

The next stage is transition. There is some general agreement that the first phase of transition occupies the time between the first month and the third to fourth month after qualification. This stage is also identified as the most difficult period of transition for newly registered nurses.

During this stage you may experience feelings of uncertainty, unpredictability and isolation, which in turn may lead to significant disruption. It may be for you that the initial excitement associated with gaining employment quickly turns to feeling unprepared for the responsibility and workload of your new role. This shift may pose numerous challenges to you both personally and professionally. During the first few weeks in the new post Gerry has been feeling overwhelmed as a result of the increase in accountability and workload. Accountability will be explored in more depth later in the chapter.

Rites of incorporation

For van Gennep, the final stage of the rites of passage was 'incorporation'. This was characterised by the individual taking up their new status and identity, and then being accepted by the group (van Gennep, 1960). This concept is particularly useful in developing a critical insight into how you may integrate into your new place of work. This stage is characterised as a relatively stable level of comfort and confidence with roles, responsibilities and routines. Gerry has spoken to other colleagues about this stage and is looking forward to feeling more confident and knowledgeable in the new post.

The process of transition

It is important for you to understand the impact that the change from student to newly registered nurse can have on you both personally and professionally. The following diagram illustrates the range of emotions that can occur when someone is working through change.

Figure 1.2 illustrates the Personal Transition Curve developed by John Fisher to describe the journey individuals go through emotionally when faced with a change. You may experience some or none of these emotions. If we look once again at Gerry's situation, the point between anxiety and happiness is where Gerry is positioned.

Figure 1.2 illustrates some of the emotions that you may experience during your transition. From looking at the diagram you may have begun to consider some of these emotions.

Activity 1.1   Decision making

Now reflect on the stage of transition you are at and position yourself on Fisher's transition curve. Consider why you have placed yourself in that position. This may be dependent on where you are in your transition journey. For example, if you are still a student you might want to think about this as you prepare for transition. Analyse the emotions that you are feeling. Consider how you will deal with this and take positive actions to develop coping strategies to ensure a smoother transition journey.

There is an outline answer at the end of the chapter.

It is important to note that although you may have identified negative emotions there is an upward curve at the end of this process. Following on from this we believe that if you can identify these emotions in yourself then this is the first step in your ability to manage the change.

We believe that it is important that you have the opportunity to discuss your transition and prepare yourself for the process. Anticipatory preparation can aid the transition whereas lack of preparation can inhibit the process and outcome, and therefore identifying the strategies that might be helpful for managing your transition may enhance the process and outcome (Meleis *et al.*, 2000). Throughout this book strategies are identified to help you to prepare for your transition.

Worthy of note is that this perceived lack of preparation is reported most often at the start of the first stage of transition. Newly registered nurses perceive lack of preparation as particularly profound at the beginning of their first stage of transition.

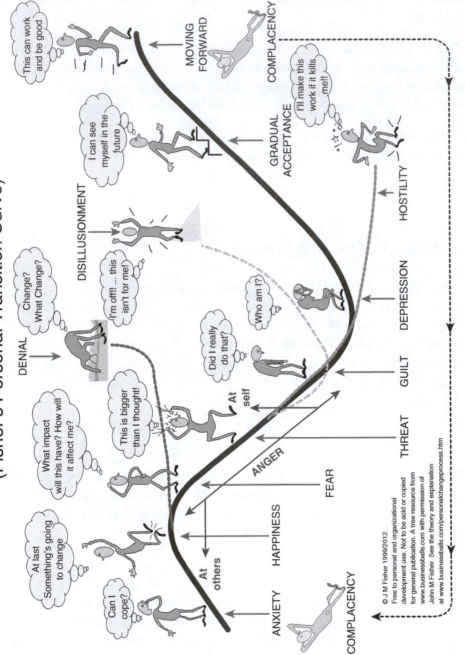

Figure 1.2 The process of transition

John Fisher (2012) (Permission for the use of this diagram has been provided by John Fisher).

Like Gerry you may feel nervous about your impending transition. By reading this chapter you will understand more about transition and you can identify that this is a usual feeling. It is important to note that you can prepare for your transition. You might want to consider forward planning. Activities to achieve this are suggested throughout this book. You can identify what you need to learn and implement into planning your development needs. If you are able to identify this process it can enable you to develop transition resilience and take control of your learning and development to enhance your experiences of transition. For example, Gerry had some concerns about the administration of medicines and therefore in the final placement implemented a personal development plan to overcome this knowledge and experience deficit. Grant and Kinman (2014) argue that resilience reflects the ability to recover from adversity, react appropriately, or bounce back when life gets tough. This can be true for newly registered nurses and we believe that you can prepare for your transition by becoming resilient to this change and developing transition resilience. We define this as the ability to cope with the anxiety and stress of transition by preparing and implementing transition-focussed personal and professional learning and development strategies. Resilience will be explored in more depth in Chapter 4.

Activities that can help and guide you to develop transition resilience are reflection, self-assessments and the creation of personal development plans that you can use as a visual plan. For example, through undertaking a range of self-assessments and formulating a Strengths, Weaknesses, Opportunities and Threats (SWOT) analysis you can be clear about your personal transition development needs and this in turn will help you to be assertive and take control of your own learning with the support of your preceptor. Further detailed information about undertaking self-assessments and formulating a SWOT analysis is explored in Chapter 2.

Accountability

One of the main challenges that you may face during your transition journey is the increase in responsibility and accountability for your actions. Indeed Gerry has recently been thinking about the increase in accountability, visualising it as an image of a big cloud stuck above the head with the word accountability written on it. Professional nursing accountability is about taking responsibility for nursing care, justifying decisions, judgements, actions and omissions. The increase in newly registered nurses' responsibility and accountability is arguably the main difference between the student and the staff nurse role (Darvill, 2013). You may perceive a shift from being a supervised individual with responsibility for your own actions to an individual not only fully accountable for your own actions, but also in some cases for the actions of others. Indeed the NMC (2015) state that nurses should be accountable for their decisions to delegate tasks and duties to other people. However, the process of adapting and coming to terms with this increased accountability is embodied in your transition experience. The increase in accountability may be particularly overwhelming and stressful.

As student nurses, it is important to be aware of the levels of responsibility required to make effective clinical judgements. You may underestimate the preparation required for your new role and need support to manage the challenges faced. This issue will be discussed in more detail later in the chapter and in Chapter 7.

As Gerry identified earlier in the chapter, at the start of transition the increase in accountability was particularly marked.

Activity 1.2   Critical thinking

Consider your own thoughts and feelings around this increase in accountability. Then summarise your previous experiences of taking responsibility for nursing care.

There is an outline answer at the end of the chapter.

This activity may have highlighted areas that will be challenging for you in relation to your increased accountability. Summarising your previous experiences may have made you aware that you can manage challenging situations in practice and have taken responsibility for your actions, it may have identified that you need to develop learning needs and goals to increase the opportunities to take responsibility. Activities relating to this are developed in Chapter 2 and 3.

Transition

In order to understand the impact of transition on you as an individual, you must first of all develop your knowledge of the underpinning theories.

Research summary

Kramer (1974) in her book *Reality Shock: Why Nurses Leave Nursing* focussed on the realities of clinical practice as manifested and dealt with by new registered nurses. Kramer coined the term 'reality shock' to describe the: *specific shock like reactions of new workers where they find themselves in a work situation for which they have spent several years preparing for which they thought they were prepared and suddenly find they are not* (p8).

More recently, Boychuk Duchscher's (2007) findings extend Kramer's work by outlining experiences of emotional, physical, intellectual, developmental and socio-cultural changes that occur within the experience of transition. She termed this 'transition shock'. Boychuk Duchscher (2007) added further insight by explaining that it was dominated by an increased awareness of accountability and a perception of being unprepared for the added responsibility of becoming a registered nurse in clinical practice. This adjustment to the new role was also correlated with inadequate and insufficient functional and emotional support and lack of confidence.

Scenario

During the first six weeks Gerry has had some opportunity to develop competency in certain job specific clinical skills. This has been a positive aspect of the transition experience and an opportunity to develop professional capability, which includes competence in a specified range of tasks, roles and jobs required of the post. However, recently the clinical area has become short staffed and Gerry is experiencing lack of support and feelings of threat and fear (see Fisher's Figure 1.2). Gerry is experiencing 'a crisis' of confidence in expectations, knowledge, skills and attitudes.

Confidence and self-efficacy

As a newly registered nurse you will often face challenges and like Gerry you may doubt your abilities. Your confidence or belief in your own abilities to deal with various situations can play a key role in not only how you feel about yourself, but also whether or not you successfully achieve your goals during your transition.

Concept summary

It is identified that confidence is a key concept in relation to transition and is closely linked to self-efficacy. Self-efficacy refers to the belief in one's own ability to succeed in a given task. Bandura (1997a) found that an individual's self-efficacy plays a major role in how goals, tasks and challenges are approached and achieved. Self-efficacy is influenced by your confidence and belief in being able to achieve your desired goals. Bandura also stated that people could be persuaded to believe that they have the skills and capabilities to succeed.

Your own responses and emotional reactions to situations will play an important role in your confidence and achievement. A lack of confidence is linked to newly registered nurses' feelings of not being prepared for their new role (Boychuk Duchscher, 2007). Professional confidence is an internal feeling of self-assurance and comfort (Crooks *et al.*, 2005). On becoming a registered nurse, you may experience a lack of confidence. It is important to know that you are not alone with this feeling. Other new nurses experience a crisis of confidence in the early stages of their transition.

When preparing for your transition to newly registered nurse, you may be able to identify goals you want to accomplish, things you would like to change, and things you would like to achieve. You should find Chapter 2 very helpful with this. However, you may also realise that putting these plans into action is not quite so simple. The following activity may help you to consider this in more depth.

Activity 1.3   Decision making

The following is a list of phrases identifying how individuals approach and achieve goals, challenges and tasks.

Identify which of these phrases below relate to you:

1.   I view challenging problems as tasks to be mastered.
2.   I develop deeper interest in the activities in which I participate.
3.   I form a stronger sense of commitment to my interests and activities.
4.   I recover quickly from setbacks and disappointments.
5.   I avoid challenging tasks.
6.   I believe that difficult tasks and situations are beyond my capabilities.
7.   I focus on personal failings and negative outcomes.
8.   I quickly lose confidence in my personal abilities.

There is an outline answer at the end of the chapter.

You may recognise that statements 1–4 indicate positive responses whereas statements 5–8 identify more negative responses. If you have chosen more of the negative responses identified then this may be an area that you need to develop. The most effective way of developing a strong sense of confidence in your ability to deal with challenging tasks and activities is by performing a task successfully; however, failing to adequately deal with a task or challenge can undermine and weaken your confidence. Sometimes nurses need confidence to say that they are not sufficiently skilled to undertake a task rather than go ahead regardless, posing risks to patient safety. So response 6 is applicable in this situation. As in the previous scenario, Gerry could do this by raising concerns and asking for guidance, help and support during this time.

Indeed, the NMC (2015) identifies that nurses should be able to recognise their limitations. Chapter 2 will enable you to undertake self-assessments and Chapter 3 formulate transition focused personal development plans to address any developmental needs you may have.

You may have witnessed other people successfully completing a task with confidence. You will have been observed by others succeeding in a task, for example by your mentor, and therefore this will have reinforced your self belief that you can achieve your goals. Getting verbal encouragement from others helps you to overcome self doubt.

On your next placement, ask your mentor to provide you with positive feedback on your successful completion of tasks. This will help you to increase your confidence.

As you approach your transition you may feel your confidence wavering and as a result experience performance anxiety and self doubt. However this lack of confidence is short lived as you develop knowledge and experience in your new role and develop a strong professional identity.

Considering that there are patterns to the way individuals develop confidence during their experiences of transition you should develop strategies for managing the roles, responsibilities and routines accompanying the change in status. Such activities include setting achievable goals, asking for feedback on performance, gaining support when faced with challenges and, perceiving your challenges as gaining knowledge and experience. Activities to help you set achievable goals will be developed further in Chapter 3.

Like Gerry it is important to acknowledge that time is a significant factor in allowing for consolidation of skills with experience to enhance confidence. Most clinical areas require completion of job specific competencies during the transition period. Gerry's confidence will increase by successfully completing these competencies with support and guidance.

Support

It is apparent that the initial stage of transition may be a time of anxiety and stress for you, and that this may be linked to your feelings of being unprepared, lacking in confidence and changes in responsibility and accountability. The need for support is a key factor that may help or hinder your experiences of transition. Chapter 7 will expand on the issue of support during your transition.

Once you qualify you will expect to be supported during your transition by a preceptor. In the UK a preceptor is defined as a registered nurse who works in the same area of practice and setting as the newly registered nurse and who is available to help, to advise and to support them (NMC, 2006). Preceptorship is defined as: *A period of structured transition for the newly registered practitioner during which he or she will be supported by a preceptor, to develop their confidence as an autonomous professional, refine skills, values and behaviours and to continue on their journey of life-long learning* (DH, 2010, p11).

Newly registered nurses benefit from a period of supported and structured preceptorship, which leads to improved recruitment and retention for the employing organisations. Transition interventions and strategies do lead to improvements in confidence and competence, job satisfaction, critical thinking and reductions in stress and anxiety for the newly qualified nurses (Whitehead *et al.*, 2013; Edwards *et al.*, 2015).

You may find that support from senior colleagues is highly valued and perceived as having a significant impact on your ability to cope with the demands of the job and an increase in confidence levels, and that it could lead to perceived stress reduction. Conversely, a perceived lack of support in the period of transition increases your anxiety and feelings of disillusionment and inadequacy. It is important that you recognise this perceived lack of support and seek help from your colleagues who can provide support to identify and address your support needs.

Anecdotally, students report that they have learned that some mentors can be relied on for support in their preparation for transition. They valued mentors who questioned them, pushed them, but did not like mentors who had too much confidence in them and expected them to be able to do everything. They benefited from being guided and supported by a 'good' mentor.

During your final placements and your preparation for transition your mentor is an important factor in your development.

Activity 1.4   Reflection

Think back to the time when you experienced the support of a mentor who you considered a role model. Define the attributes and qualities of this mentor and identify how these attributes and qualities enhanced your development.

There is an outline answer at the end of the chapter.

You may have identified that your mentor was very patient and got you involved in many activities. Your mentor may have understood your fears in relation to your transition journey. You may have felt that your mentor was honest, patient and willing to give you the most out of your placement. The mentor would contact anybody who they felt was beneficial to your learning experience. You may have built a therapeutic relationship from the beginning. Mentor support could have helped you develop qualities in becoming a better nurse.

Gerry has considered the above activity and decided that these are the qualities that a preceptor should have. You could discuss these expectations with your preceptor at the start of your transition journey.

Factors that may facilitate or inhibit your transition from student to newly registered nurse

Darvill (2013) and Croughan (2016) identified that there are factors that may facilitate or inhibit your transition from student to newly registered nurse. Therefore we feel it is important to consider them at this point. A factor that can aid your transition experience is having a supernumerary period at the start of your transition, which means that you are additional to the clinical workforce. This should include being allocated a period of time shadowing an experienced practitioner or a preceptor. This supernumerary period allows you to begin to practice and develop knowledge, skills, experience and confidence in job specific competencies in the physical presence of a supporting member of staff. This is explored further in Chapter 7.

Additionally, ensuring that you are not placed in situations beyond your confidence and competence levels without the necessary support. It is important to be allocated to a caseload whose care is within your capability as this will enable you to work independently. You can then use strategies to manage these clinical situations based on your previous knowledge, experience and skills.

Despite reaching the milestone of caring for a caseload independently, it is important for a successful transition to seek support from your colleagues. This helps you to realise that you are able to work independently, showing advancement in autonomy, knowledge, skill and experience but that you can still gain the support of others. It seems that during your transition stage, it is ideal to continue to have experienced colleagues available for support in order to have knowledge validated and to provide help and guidance (Darvill, 2013).

Other factors that may support you are:

- supportive preceptors and other staff;
- opportunity to practise skills in a supportive environment;
- education sessions including simulation practice;
- confidence increase through achievement of tasks;
- feedback on performance from preceptor;
- variance in experiences.

Factors that may challenge you:

- high staff expectations failing to acknowledge that you do not know everything;
- stress of new job;
- unsupportive preceptor;
- unrealistic personal expectations that you will be able to 'hit the ground running'.

If transition is viewed as a negative experience then this may hinder the process and your progress. It has been suggested that shadowing your preceptor and not being included as part of the workforce for a given period of time could alleviate the initial shock-like reaction. The aim of this is to facilitate your learning and practice skills without being overloaded by the overwhelming weight of responsibility that comes with managing a full clinical workload. However, you may not experience these shock-like reactions during the initial stages of your new job; they may manifest at a later stage but, with insight and incorporation of some of the elements below, this can be alleviated. Some of your initial experiences of transition may include:

- being provided with the physical presence of a supporting individual;
- being provided with a supernumerary period, which is a separate time period at the start to learn and develop job specific knowledge and skills;
- having previous knowledge, skills, experience and competencies recognised;
- undertaking an assessment of competence in job specific skills prior to working independently;
- being given feedback on job performance;
- being allocated workload based on previous experience and capability level;
- being provided with opportunities to develop your knowledge, skills and experiences;
- considering strategies for stress reduction, for example relaxation and exercise;
- developing personal, professional and academic development plans of your individual learning needs;
- networking with other newly registered practitioners;
- being given the autonomy to work independently to gain confidence through experience.

There are other influencing factors that we believe make a difference to your experiences of transition. Intrinsic and extrinsic factors such as your socio-economic background, education, upbringing, cultural background, social support, morals, values and belief systems can have significant impact on your transition. You might consider informing colleagues, family, friends, children, spouses and parents of the potential challenges you may be dealing with during the initial couple of months after you begin working as a new nurse. These could include:

- exhaustion (you may sleep a lot but don't feel rested—your sleep may be consumed with dreaming about work);
- fear of failure (you may be more defensive than usual or sensitive to critique and comments, you may have a tendency to ask questions repeatedly);

- performance anxiety (avoiding particularly difficult or new skills, avoiding patients who are ill, experiencing physical symptoms of anxiety such as sweating, racing heart, shortness of breath or inability to think/concentrate before or during a task);
- frequently changing emotions (for example laughing one minute, crying the next; you may feel anger at work or at home and be easily provoked to tears);
- low self-confidence (for example you seem to react rather than respond to comments and many comments can be taken 'personally'; you may need unusual levels of affirmation or reassurance).

The following activity may help you to consider the factors and challenges you may face.

Activity 1.5   Communication

Arrange to speak to your colleagues who have experienced transition from student to newly registered nurse and ask them what factors helped them in their first months in their new role.

As this activity is based on individual experiences there is no outline answer at the end of the chapter.

Your colleagues may have shared their experiences of transition which are similar to the challenges identified in this chapter, however you could have also discussed with them the factors that assisted them during that time and consider whether these would be helpful to you. Here are some tips to help you survive your first year and be a successful nurse:

- be organised – try a few different methods and choose one that works for you, then keep it consistent;
- prioritise your workload and ensure all your tasks are complete. Recognise that there are also some that can be delayed;
- never hesitate to ask questions;
- accept help from others;
- practise efficiency;
- be proactive;
- make friends with your new colleagues;
- make time for a break;
- accept you might make mistakes but report them if you do;
- keep in contact with others who are also experiencing the transition;
- understand it gets better.

Following the initial phase of transition, the second or intermediate phase usually occurs between three to four months and six months of the newly registered nurses' experience. During this time Gerry noticed a consistent and rapid advancement in thinking, knowledge, skill and competency level. It seems that this period of time is dominated by learning to establish your place in the organisation. Nurses report that they are able to integrate the knowledge developed during their undergraduate programme with practical skills they had developed since qualifying (Clark and Holmes, 2007). During this phase it is likely that your confidence will increase. In addition, this stage is about fitting in, learning the rules and your position in the hierarchy. However, you are still in a period of transition and must be able to recognise your limitations. Avoid being placed in positions beyond your competence without the necessary support. If you are allocated to responsibilities that you feel are beyond your capability and competence then it is important to raise this with your preceptor rather than undertaking the care. Try to situate yourself in familiar practice situations during these initial stages to allow for consistency, familiarity and predictability within your level of competence, skill, cognitive ability and experience. This will help in alleviating anxiety.

You may notice that by six months you should begin to adapt more readily to the 'real-world' of practice and be able to implement the necessary knowledge and skills for the post.

Meleis *et al.* (2000) suggest that the end of an experience of transition is marked by the extent to which individuals demonstrate mastery of the skills and behaviour needed to manage their situations. Newly registered nurses towards the end of the first year are able to demonstrate capability in their role although there is some debate as to whether there is a full incorporation (Darvill, 2013).

However, there is recognition that there is still a long way to go and still more to learn and achieve, You may still experience feelings of uncertainty and still feel new. One of the emotions identified in Fisher's diagram is complacency. Fisher states that if you are feeling complacent you feel that you have survived the change and moved into your 'comfort zone'. You may feel that you know the right decisions to make and can predict future events with a high degree of certainty. However, this may be a problematic situation as you may not be able to identify potential risks. It is important that you recognise this complacency and it may be that you need to set yourself new challenges and new goals for your future career development. Chapter 8 deals with this issue in more detail.

Chapter summary

This chapter has defined the concept of transition. Transition is a process of how final year nursing students in becoming registered nurses adjust to the responsibilities of this new role. We have provided you with the opportunity to reflect on your thoughts, feelings and perceptions of your personal transition journey. We have identified some common factors that you may find challenging in moving to being a newly registered nurse, including the increase in accountability, the possibility of wavering confidence levels and the need for support. Transitions are experienced in a series of stages with a beginning, middle and an end. The stages of transition have been explained, starting with separation, which begins with a realisation of the impending change in status. The transition stage can be a time of anxiety and stress, and this can lead to perceived feelings of being unprepared. However, incorporation into the new role can be mastered with a gradual acceptance of the role and an increase in knowledge and skill level. Preparation for transition is crucial to develop transition resilience.

Activities: brief outline answers

Activity 1.1 Decision making (page 11)

An example of where you have positioned yourself may be disillusionment. If you are feeling disillusioned because your core beliefs and values do not seem to fit with your new position, you may then acknowledge these feelings and ask for help and support from your colleagues and consider how you can deal with these feelings. Conversely, you may experience gradual acceptance, which includes you beginning to make sense of your environment and of your place within the organisation. You are beginning to get some validation of your thoughts and actions and can see that where you are going is right. This could be the start of managing your control over the change and seeing some successes. This links in with an increasing level of self-confidence.

Activity 1.2 Critical thinking (page 14)

For the first part of this activity you may have identified that you have concerns about the increase in accountability. You may be worried about making mistakes, finding decision making challenging and have concerns about being responsible for your own actions and the actions of others. You may have concerns regarding your leadership and management skills, case load management, time management, dealing with challenging situations including breaking bad news, communicating with interprofessional teams, delegation, medication administration, prioritising care and decision making skills.

Your answer might have considered these areas where you have taken responsibility:

- managing a group of patients;
- time management;
- communicating with other health professionals;
- delegation;
- clinical skills;
- assessment skills;
- managing your own learning;
- organisational skills;
- working with others and their various roles.

By summarising these responsibilities you will have identified where you have taken responsibility for nursing care.

Activity 1.3 Decision making (page 16)

Your responses to these questions may identify whether you have a strong sense of self-efficacy or a weak sense of self-efficacy (lack of confidence) in your abilities. In reference to Gerry's situation, Gerry has identified phrases 1, 2, 3 and 8 as relevant. Gerry views challenging problems as tasks to be mastered, has developed a deeper interest in job specific activities and formed a stronger sense of commitment to interests and activities; however Gerry has lost confidence in personal abilities. If you find yourself in a similar situation to Gerry's then it is important to raise your concerns and ask for help and support.

Activity 1.4 Reflection (page 18)

Your answer might consider an effective role model to be someone who:

- is approachable;
- maintains high standards of care;
- is caring, confident and positive;
- is knowledgeable;
- is passionate about learning;
- understands the student's roles and responsibilities and the stage of nurse education programme training;
- is willing and desires to be a mentor;
- is approachable.

See Croughan's work (2016) for further information.

Further reading

Croughan, CE (2016) *Student nurses' preparation and negotiation of transition to the Registered Nurse role. Are there any factors that influence or inhibit this successful negotiation and transition? A systematic review.* Unpublished MSc thesis. University of Salford. http://usir.salford.ac.uk/38397/

In this literature review you can read the evidence to identify factors that negotiate the preparation and transition from student nurse to the registered nurse role.

Darvill, A (2013) *A qualitative study into the experiences of newly qualified children's nurses during their transition into children's community nursing teams.* Unpublished PhD thesis. University of Salford. http://usir.salford.ac.uk/29369/

This research with newly registered nurses will help you to understand factors that can support an ideal transition experience.

Darvill, A, Fallon, D and Livesley, J (2014) A different world? The transition experiences of newly qualified children's nurses taking up first destination posts within children's community nursing teams. *Issues in Comprehensive Paediatric Nursing*, 37(1): 6–24.

This article explains more about the challenges and inhibitors to a successful transition for newly registered nurses.

Morrell, N and Ridgway, V (2014) Are we preparing student nurses for their final placement? *British Journal of Nursing*, 23(10): 518–23.

This research illuminates student nurses' perceptions of preparedness for final practice placement, and to ascertain factors that supported and hindered preparation for final placement practice.

Philips, C, Estermann, A and Kenny, A (2015) The theory of organisational socialisation and its potential for improving transition experiences for new graduate nurses. *Nurse Education Today*, 35: 118–24.

This Australian study of newly qualified graduate nurses highlights that orientation throughout the first year of practice, allocation of patient responsibilities reflecting a level commensurate with a beginning skill set to meet care needs, and feedback to improve confidence and competence in practice enhance transition experiences.

Zamanzadeh, V, Jasemi, V, Valizadeh, L, Keogh, B and Taleghani, B (2015) Lack of preparation: Iranian nurses' experiences during transition from college to clinical practice. *Journal of Professional Nurse*, 31: 365–73.

This Iranian study indicates that newly registered nurses were not well prepared to assume their clinical roles. This study makes suggestions that you can consider when preparing for your transition.

Useful websites

http://nursingthefuture.ca/index

This website Nursing the Future (NTF) was inspired by the research and study of Dr Judy Boychuk Duchscher. Its aim is to support and guide the newest members of the nursing profession as they move from the role of nursing student into the world of professional nursing practice.

www.businessballs.com/personalchangeprocess.htm

www.c2d.co.uk/techniques/process-of-transition/

The above two web resources provide a more detailed account of John Fisher's personal transition curve.

www.youtube.com/watch?v=xSn2qqmcwaA

This YouTube clip is by Nurse Theorist, Afaf Ibrahim Meleis speaking about her work on transition.

Chapter 2

Self-assessment of knowledge, skills and attitudinal values through critical reflection

Denise Major

Standards

NMC Standards for Pre-registration Nursing Education

As this chapter is concerned with self-awareness of the nurse's ability to develop competence in all competencies for entry to the register, its underlying principles relate to all four domains of the competencies.

Especially competence 4 of domain 4:

> *All nurses must be self-aware and recognise how their own values, principles and assumptions may affect their practice. They must maintain their own personal and professional development, learning from experience, through supervision, feedback, reflection and evaluation.*

Essential Skills Clusters

This chapter will address the following essential skills clusters:

Cluster: Care, compassion and communication

1.   As partners in the care process, people can trust a newly registered graduate nurse to provide collaborative care based on the highest standards, knowledge and competence.

1.9. Is self-aware and self-confident, knows own limitations and is able to take appropriate action.

Cluster: Organisational aspects of care

12. People can trust the newly registered graduate nurse to respond to their feedback and a wide range of other sources to learn, develop and improve services.

12.6. Actively responds to feedback.

12.8. As an individual team member and team leader, actively seeks and learns from feedback to enhance care and own and others' professional development.

14. People can trust the newly registered graduate nurse to be an autonomous and confident member of the multi-disciplinary or multi agency team and to inspire confidence in others.

14.7. Challenges the practice of self and others across the multi-professional team.

15. People can trust the newly registered graduate nurse to safely delegate to others and to respond appropriately when a task is delegated to them.

15.5. Recognises and addresses deficits in knowledge and skill in self and others and takes appropriate action.

Cluster: Medicines management

38. People can trust the newly registered graduate nurse to administer medicines safely and in a timely manner, including controlled drugs.

Chapter aims

After reading this chapter, you will be able to appreciate the value of self-assessment in facilitating your professional development, which may include:

- choosing transition-focussed self-assessment tools to assess your current stage of development towards achievement of: the NMC competencies for registration (NMC, 2010), abiding by the NMC (2015) Code;
- undertaking, and recording, a personal, professional and academic self-assessment of your knowledge, skills and attitudinal values in relation to your transition from student nurse to newly registered nurse;
- constructing a composite SWOT or SNOB analysis (Humphrey, 2005; Sykes, 2012) of the findings from your self-assessments, in readiness for making transition-focussed personal development plans (Major, 2015).

Introduction

The chapter will begin by introducing a student nurse scenario and a concept summary of self-assessment as the foundation for knowing yourself at your current point in your transition journey. After this foundation, we will explore how to select self-assessment tools relevant to your transition from student to newly registered nurse. There are activities for selecting the tools and constructing your own self-assessment recording sheets. After undertaking your own self-assessments, the chapter will guide you through constructing an analysis of your self-assessment findings to identify your strengths, weaknesses and learning needs, learning opportunities and barriers or threats to your learning. This analysis can then be used for building transition-focussed personal development plans (TFPDPs) to reach the desired new identity of newly registered nurse.

Let us now introduce student nurse Bobby, whose transition journey is the focus of this chapter.

Scenario

Bobby is a student nurse entering the final year of the nursing degree course. Bobby has been achieving fairly good grades of around 58–62 per cent in academic work and is determined to improve on this in order to complete the degree course with a minimum classification of 2:1. So far, Bobby has achieved all of the professional practice learning outcomes at the first attempt, with good mentor and patient feedback. Bobby is hoping to apply for a job at the local children's ward.

Bobby contacted the personal tutor for help with making plans for achieving personal final-year aspirations, as Bobby recognises that it is going to be a busy year and feels the need to be well organised. Bobby is both excited and apprehensive about making the transition from student to newly registered nurse.

Bobby's situation is common to many final year students. Therefore, we will use Bobby's scenario to provide context for the self-assessments that any student could undertake as a baseline for setting TFPDPs.

What is self-assessment and why use it?

Concept summary: self-assessment

Self-assessment for a final year student nurse entails undertaking a critical reflection on where you are now in relation to the expected professional standards of knowledge, skills and attitudinal values that you must acquire, and achieve competence in performing, by the end of your nursing education.

Self-assessment provides a personal awareness of one's abilities and learning needs in order to plan to progress through one's career in the profession, not only before, but also after, Registration. The undergraduate period is an ideal time to start rehearsal of these skills while you have the continual support and supervision of your academic and practice tutors. Keep in mind that this transition is a journey, managing the gradual change in your learning and your role identity from student to newly registered nurse. As an active part of that journey, these self-assessments will provide you with information for making sound, evaluative judgements of what knowledge, skills and values you already have. Knowing your strengths through self-assessment will provide you with personal confidence to extend your learning for those elements needing development. Self-assessments will help you to internalise the psychological progression of your thoughts, feelings and values since starting your nurse education. Learning to make sound, evaluative judgements will also help you to determine the usefulness of the resources that you are able to access, and determine the progress you are making in your personal, professional and academic development towards registration.

Context summary: self-assessment as the foundation of knowing yourself

The self-assessments described in this chapter will help you to 'know yourself' by establishing your current role and identity as a professional. Transition is a period of psychological adjustment, as well as a time to consolidate the skills needed to perform the newly registered nurse role. Successful transition requires a sense of mastery of changed events and a re-orientation of self-identity. This re-orientation of self-identity requires thinking deeply about yourself. Establishing a current self-identity through self-assessment, and comparing this to the desired new professional identity written in the NMC competencies and Code (NMC, 2015) will help you to define your personal, professional and academic development needs for this preparation for transition year.

These development needs will provide the basis for goal setting and personal development planning focussed specifically on your transition towards the new personal, professional and academic self. Carrying out your development plans will involve a period of acquisition of knowledge, social and professional support, and learning ways to adapt to the forthcoming new role. The heightened self-awareness and increased self-efficacy, which comes from an organised way of learning, contrasts greatly with going to placement, or undertaking academic work, with little preparation and planning. Following a mechanistic model of learning knowledge and skills, without any underpinning independence in study, organisational ability, or resilience during times of demanding professional work could leave you ill-equipped to maintain a fast-paced, evolving career.

Therefore, using active self-assessments and purposeful learning throughout the transition journey will ensure that you arrive at your new professional identity with secure, competent knowledge, skills and attitudinal values for the role, as well as having the psychological re-orientation to think and react as a newly registered nurse.

If you are feeling that this transition from your known world of student to the expected world of a newly registered nurse is rather daunting and a huge challenge, undertake Activity 2.1 to see how a well-known public figure has made a life-changing transition.

Activity 2.1   Reflection

Watch the following YouTube clip and press coverage which shows racing driver Alex Zanadi achieving his goal of being a successful Paralympian competitor after a near fatal Formula One car racing accident.

www.huffingtonpost.co.uk/entry/channel-4-the-last-leg-alex-brooker-paralympics-alex-zanardi-medal_uk_57dbb555e4b028e52a1025ed

Consider how Alex Zanadi had to reassess all of his abilities and set himself incremental goals of achievement to win Paralympian Gold when his life changed from the role he was used to performing.

An outline of what you might have considered is given at the end of the chapter.

Consider how you now feel in relation to the forthcoming changes in your professional career.

From undertaking Activity 2.1 you may recognise the physical, emotional and social impact that life transitions have on us. Having this recognition helps us to appreciate that the transition journey really does require us to spend time in reflective thought and purposeful actions, in order to come through the transition with a heightened understanding and adaptation to our changed situation. It also requires gradual steps of change, and learning, in order to reach the final goals of the new identity. You will read in Chapter 3 about using reflective models to make sense of significant events in your practice and personal life. These deep, meaningful insights may have provided evidence of the need to analyse further your specific strengths and learning needs in the transition towards Registration. This chapter will lead you through transition-focussed self-assessments, which can be accompanied by continued structured reflection to provide an overall understanding of your transition journey.

Your own professional transition journey towards newly registered nurse may or may not feel as important and intense to you as Zanadi's journey did to him. However, your personal ownership of your journey will still be key to your success of arriving ready to fulfil your role and drive your career as a registered nurse. Just as Zanadi took control of his journey to a new identity with the support of those who could help him to redefine his role identity as a top-performing racing driver, you will need to take control and seek support, to learn to perform your redefined nursing role at Registration.

As Zanadi inspired Brooker, you too may have your own personal and professional role models who will inspire you to achieve your goals. However, you will need to be fully aware of your starting point in relation to those goals, otherwise it can be very difficult to set realistic, manageable objectives along the way, in order to reach that final goal of registration. Self-assessment will help you to determine your starting point of where you are now in your professional journey towards registration, so that you can make and implement your own personalised TFPDPs. Table 2.1 outlines a common format for a Personal Development Plan and illustrates how self-assessment through critical reflection forms the first stage of writing this.

Constructing the entire, detailed plan will be addressed in Chapter 3. For now, we just need to concentrate on the self-assessment aspects.

Selecting self-assessment tools relevant to your transition from student to newly registered nurse

You should already be familiar with the practice and academic requirements for nursing registration, as the Nursing and Midwifery Council (NMC, 2010) competencies are contained within your practice-based assessments and the academic level required for registration is reflected in your university's final year academic grading criteria. Your self-assessments should therefore take into account both the practice and academic aspects of your learning in relation to all of the competency domains in the NMC Standards (NMC, 2010).

When undertaking a self-assessment, it is so important to identify not only your learning needs and weaknesses, but also your abilities and strengths; academic strengths,

Working from left to right to complete the content for each column heading, will provide logical sequencing and an easy-to-read progress chart.					
Self-assessment	Setting SMART learning objectives	Resources, actions and strategies	Sources of evidence	Review date	Results of review/ evaluation of progress
Strengths, weaknesses and learning needs identified from personal, professional and academic self-assessments of knowledge, skills and attitudinal values					

Table 2.1   TFPDP outline template, showing self-assessment as the first stage

professional strengths, personal strengths and personal qualities. These all help you to learn, support you in times of stress and help you to gain access to learning opportunities in clinical practice and university. Don't underestimate the personal qualities that you already have, and equally, don't shy away from personal and social development needs; they are just as important as academic or professional learning needs in keeping you and your family well and in harmony with supporting your endeavours to become a newly registered nurse.

There are various self-assessment tools available to help you to self-assess and make 'value judgements' about yourself. However, there is no exact number of self-assessments to be undertaken, nor is the list of suggested self-assessment tools exhaustive, so be reassured that if you find other tools that objectively suit your purpose, go ahead and use them, as it is your decision as to which tools will be most useful to you. The sum total of all of your self-assessments can be quite enlightening, so long as you are honest about your achievements and use recognised assessment criteria against which to make your evaluative judgements. As it is often difficult to be totally objective about yourself, it is crucial that you include the evidence for why you are making those judgements about your knowledge, performance and attitudinal characteristics. Activity 2.2 will help you to think about what self-assessment tools and evidence of achievements can be useful to you.

Activity 2.2 Critical thinking

Have a look at Table 2.2 and list all of those self-assessment tools that are relevant to your own transition journey from student to newly registered nurse.

Sometimes you will need to be courageous in choosing a self-assessment tool that you don't feel comfortable with, or that you feel that you 'don't like', either because it causes you some personal disquiet or, perhaps you do not understand how to use it. You can read more about the tools by using the references in Table 2.2 or the 'useful websites' at the end of the chapter.

Consider carefully what 'evidence of achievement' will actually give you the information that you need, in order to know about your personal, professional and academic knowledge, skills and attitudinal values.

At the end of the chapter, you can see an outline answer of the tools that Bobby might have chosen to use, and reasons for their choice.

You could now construct your own table of the tools and evidence that you would use for your self-assessments. *Your answers may be different to Bobby's, but that is to be expected, because of the individual nature of each person's own transition journey.*

Having chosen your self-assessment tools, we can now move on to considering how we can use these tools to undertake a self-assessment.

	Personal self-assessment tools.	Professional self-assessment tools. Several of these contain knowledge, skills and attitudinal values.	Academic self-assessment tools.
Knowledge	Personal knowledge about how to access learning resources within the university and placements.	NMC generic and field-specific competencies and essential skills clusters (NMC, 2010). Standards for competence for registered nurses (NMC, 2014). Ten commitments for nursing (National Health Service England, 2016/05). Inventory of learning needs (Major, 2010, p189). Knowledge and skills framework outlines for nursing posts (Royal College of Nursing, 2005). NHS leadership model self-assessment tool (NHS Leadership Academy 2013, 2015). Team roles (Belbin, 1981).	Learning styles inventories (Fleming and Mills, 1992; Honey and Mumford, 2000). University level 6 and level 7 assessment grading criteria. Making the most of feedback (Sykes, 2012). Framework for higher education qualifications bachelors level grading criteria (QAA, 2008). Cognitive taxonomy of educational objectives: (Bloom and Krathwohl, 1956; Krathwohl and Anderson, 2010).
Skills	Personal qualities for learning (Major, 2010, p207).		Psychomotor domain taxonomy of learning objectives: (Dave, 1970; Harrow, 1972; Simpson, 1972).
Attitudinal values	Johari Window (Luft, 1969). Personality-type questionnaire (Myers and Briggs, 1962). Emotional intelligence scales (Schutte, Malouff and Bhullar, 2009). Self-efficacy scales (Chen, Gully and Eden, 2001). Fisher's personal transition curve (Fisher, 2012).	Johari Window (Luft, 1969). De Bono's (2016) *Six Thinking Hats* for decision making.	Affective domain taxonomy of learning objectives: (Bloom, Krathwhol and Masia, 1964).
Possible sources of evidence of achievements	Personal structured reflections. Verbal comments from friends and colleagues.	Practice assessment documents. Personal Development record. Reflections on significant events in practice.	Academic assessment feedback and marks or grades achieved. Reflections on academic progress.

Table 2.2   Possible transition-focussed self-assessment tools and sources of evidence for your achievements

Selecting and constructing self-assessment recording sheets

Many of the self-assessment tools have their own in-built self-assessment recording sheets; however, some do not. Therefore, like Bobby, if you choose to use those without, it will be very useful to you to be able to construct your own recording sheets. There are some examples in Figures 2.1 to 2.3 of self-assessment recording sheets across the Personal, Professional and Academic aspects.

Personal self-assessment

The self-assessment recording tool in Figure 2.1 is written using a five-point Likert scale (Likert, 1932), to measure the respondent's attitudes, values or beliefs towards the content. Figure 2.1 has been completed with some examples of Bobby's possible responses and their evidence.

A Likert scale helps the user to make a value judgement about how the issue being assessed applies to themselves. Although the Likert scale relies on a personal, subjective viewpoint, in Figure 2.1 a column has been added for evidence to verify the responses. Thus, users are required to question themselves; for example, 'How do I know that I am proactive?' Providing this evidence reduces the subjectivity of the responses.

The content of Figure 2.1 was constructed from Major's (2010) research, where 'Managing one's own learning' emerged as a theme from the conversations with final year students. They recognised that having certain personal qualities helped them to communicate better with their clinical practice mentors and supervisors, so that they could explain what they were particularly interested in learning and get the most benefit from the learning opportunities that were available.

Raising your own self-awareness of how your personal qualities for learning are developed, or need developing, can provide reassurance, or direction for improvement. Those students who have well-developed personal qualities are obviously better equipped for learning than those who still need to develop them. In Activity 2.2, Bobby recognised the development of personal qualities as an important learning objective, to enable a purposefully facilitated transition. The personal qualities needed for managing your own learning are also valuable precursors to the personal qualities needed for leadership (NHS Leadership Academy, 2013).

You might like to read more about 'personal qualities' from the further reading list at the end of the chapter.

Strongly linked to personal qualities for learning is the notion of 'self-efficacy' previously discussed in Chapter 1. Self-efficacy is not just about being an effective organiser of your studies, it also contains elements of emotional intelligence that will provide the internal psychological support needed to build the confidence to try new situations

	Strongly agree	Agree	Neither agree nor disagree	Disagree	Strongly disagree	Evidence for this perceived level of achievement
1. I am proactive	X					I make learning plans for my placements.
2. I am self-aware		X				I read feedback and discuss it with tutors.
3. I am self-directed	X					I look ahead in my development record to see what is required each semester.
4. I am resourceful		X				I ask for help, use library and online resources.
5. I am motivated	X					I want to finish on time with a 2:1 I have good academic feedback.
6. I am able to drive the process of learning		X				I use structured reflections on personal, professional and academic significant events. I discuss learning opportunities and my needs in each placement. I book assignment supervision.
7. I am a good communicator		X				I use voicemail, email and personal contact. My mentors say my record keeping in practice meets NMC standards.
8. I am assertive			X			I am just a bit wary of some new skills: Mentor feedback regarding reluctance to undertake new clinical skills.

Figure 2.1   Major's (2010) personal qualities as a self-assessment tool

with positivity. If you can increase your self-efficacy, your personal qualities for learning will also increase, thus helping you to get the most out of available learning opportunities in university and placements.

The self-efficacy recording sheet in Figure 2.2 uses the same Likert scale self-assessment tool as the personal qualities self-assessment. It has again been completed with some possible answers from Bobby.

Derived from Chen, Gully and Eden's (2001) new general self-efficacy scale, with the addition of an 'Evidence of achievement' column, the self-assessment tool in Figure 2.2 was included within Major's (2015) follow-on research. Final year student nurses reported a significant increase in their personal self-efficacy when they engaged in active learning, using critical, reflective self-assessment as a foundation for writing their TFPDPs (Major, 2015).

The items below are from Chen, Gully and Eden, 2001: p79 Appendix.	Strongly agree	Agree	Neither agree nor disagree	Disagree	Strongly disagree	Evidence of achievement
"1. I will be able to achieve most of the goals I have set for myself."			X			I usually set short interim goals to achieve the overall outcomes required. This year feels a bit overwhelming so I am not sure, but I will use this previous strategy.
"2. When facing difficult tasks, I am certain that I will accomplish them."			X			Unsure how difficult final year will be. Achieved well in some intense placement situations (see mentor feedback).
"3. In general, I think that I can obtain outcomes that are important to me."		X				I work hard and have achieved all PDPs so far.
"4. I believe I can succeed at most any endeavour to which I set my mind."		X				I have passed all of my assignments at first attempt so far. I will try hard for a 2:1 in final year.
"5. I will be able to successfully overcome many challenges."		X				I know what is expected in NMC competencies.
"6. I am confident that I can perform effectively on many different tasks."			X			Not sure, but I will try. I usually do succeed. Finding it hard to manage several demands from home, university and practice.
"7. Compared to other people, I can do most tasks very well."			X			I am pretty average compared to peers and their feedback.
"8. Even when things are tough, I can perform quite well."		X				I have worked with determination and always seek support.

Figure 2.2   Construction of a recording sheet for your personal self-efficacy

Source: Major, 2015: adapted from Chen, Gully and Eden, 2001.

Being active and in control of your own situated learning is paramount to managing your own transition journey amidst the turmoil that transition brings. Developing your personal qualities and self-efficacy will enable you to actively seize opportunities to learn and work in partnership with all of those people who support your learning journey. This sense of belonging, and control, will give you a much stronger sense of achievement, rather than the uncertainty of just letting things happen and hoping others will provide for you.

Professional self-assessment

The NMC competencies (NMC, 2010) provide the essential, definitive learning outcomes for student nurses in order to gain registration. However, there is no specific self-assessment tool built into it. Your practice assessment document may have its own self-assessment recording tool. If not, Figure 2.3 provides an example of a partially completed self-assessment recording sheet for two competency statements, one generic and one field competence. Be sure to use the full field standard for your own field of nursing. The example in Figure 2.3 applies only to Bobby's scenario – the Children's and Young People's field; the other fields have their own specific content.

You could construct this table to include any, or all, of the NMC competencies.

For clarity of reading in this example, the table is only partially filled in; however, the self-assessment should be worked across all knowledge, skills and attitudinal values boxes for each of the competencies that you include.

Although students must attain all of the NMC competencies by the end of their nursing education, there are certain competencies that final year student nurses often consider to be priority learning objectives as they approach newly registered nurse status. For example, Bobby's self-assessment in Activity 2.1 recognised that: *This year I have to be able to lead the team for Registration competence and my new job.*

Final placement students in Major's (2010) research said that, while completing their required NMC competencies, concentrating effort on those learning needs that were particularly significant to themselves gained them a great sense of competence, confidence and satisfaction when they had achieved them. Their main priorities were skills in management, leadership, teaching, decision making and working autonomously. They differentiated management experiences as management of themselves, management of patient care, organisation of the ward routine, leadership, and management of the staff team (Major, 2010).

Leadership and management skills are summarised in the competencies within the NMC (2010) domain 'Leadership, Management and Team-working' and should be used within your NMC self-assessment. For a more in-depth leadership self-assessment, the NHS Leadership Model will provide you with a ready-made self-assessment recording sheet (NHS Leadership Academy, 2015b).

You will see that Bobby already aspires to a specific specialty of nursing care for the newly registered nurse post, and will therefore make a self-assessment against the job description specific to that post. If you do not know which specialty you are aiming for,

NMC Competency Statements		Domain 1. **Professional Values** **Generic standard for** **competence:** **All nurses must act** **first and foremost to** **care for and protect** **the public …**	Domain 1. **Field Standard 2.** **All nurses must practice in a holistic, non-** **judgemental, caring and sensitive manner …** 2.1 Children's nurses must recognise that all children and young people have the right to be safe, enjoy life and reach their potential. They must practise in a way that recognises, respects and responds to the individuality of every child and young person.
	Self-assessment element		
Knowledge **Assessment:** **Cognitive** **Domain**	I know	I know about safe- guarding principles	
	I don't know	Local policy	
	I need to know	Local policy in placement 7, as this is the area I want to work in when newly Registered	
	Evidence for this current knowledge	reflection Year 2, semester 2.	
Skills **Assessment:** **Psychomotor** **Domain**	I can	Recognise causes of concern and report them accurately, verbally	
	I can't	I have never been involved in a safeguarding case conference	
	I need to be able to	Accurately write safeguarding accounts and explain them to other members of the MDT	
	Evidence for this current skills ability	Mentor endorsement of competence in Practice assessment document Year 2 semester 2.	
Attitudinal **Values** **Assessment:** **Affective** **Domain**	What do I feel about this aspect? What are my attitudinal values towards this?		As a Children's and Young People's nursing student, I always try to be non-judgemental towards parents when there is suspicion of possible safeguarding issues. I recognise the difficulties of parenting and the challenges which children bring to the parenting relationship. However, my first priority is to the child to make them feel welcome, valued and safe. I would listen, record and report objectively anything that they share with me. I will engage them in purposeful play appropriate to their developmental age and stage.
	What professional values should I be upholding for this aspect?		As a priority, recognise and protect children from harm at all times, through team working. Respect individuals' lifestyle choices while seizing opportunities for promoting parenting skills and communication between parents and children wherever possible.
	What is my evidence for my current attitudinal values?		I have seen several cases of mistaken, and some cases of confirmed, ill-treatment of children.

Figure 2.3 Construction of a self-assessment sheet for two of the NMC competencies
for registration (NMC, 2010) (professional domain)

you could assess yourself against the general descriptions of registered nurse posts and person specifications contained within the Department of Health's National Health Service Knowledge and Skills Framework (DoH, 2004), the Royal College of Nursing (RCN) descriptions of Nursing posts (RCN, 2005) and various NHS job advertisements. Part of your self-assessment may also include assessment of, and gaining feedback on, your interview skills. Your university student careers services and placements may provide this support.

Academic self-assessment

Your academic work will be graded at least at Bachelor's level during your final year (Quality Assurance Agency (QAA), 2008, p18), as this is the minimum academic level that the NMC will allow for registration.

Your feedback from assignments, when compared to your university grade descriptors and the QAA standards, will provide the evidence of your academic level in relation to your professional practice. This self-assessment will enable you to determine whether you need to improve your academic learning levels or learning abilities.

Being able to understand how you learn can help you to deliberately access learning materials that suit your personal learning styles and provide insight into whether you need to expand these. See Bobby's example in the feedback to Activity 2.1 about undertaking a learning styles questionnaire, such as the Honey and Mumford (2000) inventory, or Fleming and Mills' (1992) VARK assessment.

The three domains of Bloom's (1956) taxonomy, cognitive, psychomotor and affective, and the more recent revisions, are useful indicators for self-assessment of your current level of academic and professional skills achievements.

The three domains cannot really be viewed separately from each other, as all of your cognitive academic knowledge and your psychomotor skills learning are also affected by your affective, or attitudinal, values. The domains are expressed in increasing levels of complexity and you are aiming to achieve the highest level in all domains by the time of registration.

The self-effacement that comes from undertaking self-assessments is not easy; looking at ourselves, our personal qualities and how others see us can be quite unnerving. Some students choose to use the Johari window exercise (Chapman, 1995–2014) as assessment of personal qualities and relationships. For a more insightful experience of your professional abilities, be sure to ask your nursing colleagues for their evaluative feedback, rather than just using the exercise with personal friends.

Once we have some more insight into ourselves, through our own and others' assessments of our knowledge, skills and attitudinal values, there is often a feeling of obligation to improve where necessary. This obligation to improve should actually be very liberating and an exciting challenge, as it has the potential to help us succeed with things that may have previously been difficult for us.

The recording tools, whether they are in-built to the self-assessment tools, or self-constructed, will provide you with an easy-to-read account of your own personal self-assessments, so that you can go on to analyse your findings.

Undertaking the self-assessments

Activity 2.3   Critical reflection

If you have not undertaken any self-assessments yet, you should now have the information needed to try undertaking them.

Undertake your self-assessments, using each of the self-assessment tools which you selected in Activity 2.2. Remember to use the corresponding self-assessment recording sheets by obtaining any that are commercially available, or by making your own, such as suggested in Figures 2.1, 2.2 and 2.3. Be sure to include your evidence for the responses you give, as this will give validity to your findings.

As your self-assessments are personal to you, there is no outline answer at the end of the chapter. Figures 2.1 and 2.2 provide some possible responses, but be reassured that everyone's self-assessments will be different in their findings and may be constructed in their own creative manner.

Keep your self-assessment records safe, so that you can go on to analysing the findings after the next explanation.

The set of self-assessments that you have undertaken in Activity 2.3 might seem to be quite complex and you may be wondering how many self-assessments are needed. So long as you have used sufficient tools to assess knowledge, skills and attitudinal values for all three aspects of your development, personal, professional and academic, the assessment findings will provide sufficient information to make a comprehensive, systematic analysis covering all aspects of your transition journey requirements.

Every person's experience of transition from student nurse to newly registered nurse is their own individual journey, so don't be surprised if your findings are different to those of your friends and colleagues, as you will all have had different life journeys and professional experiences during your time as a student nurse. The need for change from student orientation to newly registered nurse orientation will have a different magnitude for each person. The self-assessment is going to lead onto a composite overall analysis of your strengths, your weaknesses and your learning needs. Your analysis will help you to know your current self and abilities in comparison to the required attributes of the role you are preparing yourself for.

Constructing an analysis of your strengths, weaknesses and learning needs from your self-assessments

All of your self-assessment findings can be recorded in one coherent analysis, such as a SWOT (strengths, weaknesses, opportunities and threats), or SNOB (strengths, needs, opportunities and barriers) analysis table (Tables 2.3 and 2.4).

Strengths	Weaknesses
Opportunities	Threats

Table 2.3   A SWOT analysis table

Strengths	Needs
Opportunities	Barriers

Table 2.4   A SNOB analysis table

SWOT has been proven to be a useful developmental, results-oriented strategic planning tool, used extensively in business management, and has gained a place at the forefront of many assessment and planning situations in nursing. The SNOB adaptation presents a more personalised, rather than business orientated, model to help individuals review and plan their abilities and learning as a part of personal career development planning. Which of these two formats you choose will be your personal choice; either one will provide you with a clear analysis of your current progress in clinical practice, at university and at home. Activity 2.4 will help you to make your SWOT or SNOB analysis from your self-assessments, from which you can communicate your learning needs to your academic and practice supervisors and mentors.

Activity 2.4   Reflection and critical thinking

1. Decide which format you are going to use and construct your SWOT or SNOB analysis table with sufficient space to make several entries in each box.
2. Examine each of your self-assessments in turn. Consider what they are telling you about your strengths and weaknesses, or needs. Write down the common themes that are starting to emerge across all of them.

(Continued)

(Continued)

3. Record the common themes of strengths and weaknesses, or needs in the appropriate boxes of your SWOT or SNOB table. Be sure to add which sources of evidence each theme came from.

A discussion of the themes you might find is given at the end of the chapter.

An example of a completed SWOT analysis that could be constructed from Bobby's self-assessments can be seen in Table 2.5, but first we need to consider the content of the final two boxes.

Activity 2.5   Reflection and critical thinking

Look at the opportunities to learn in the SWOT or SNOB analysis – think again about anything that may be an opportunity in your forthcoming clinical placements or university, but that you may not have accessed, such as talking to patients' parents, friends, or relatives as a vast source of information about social, psychological and physical needs; or perhaps accessing the university's student support service for study skills, presentation skills, academic writing, library skills, interviewing skills, financial advice, or counselling.

Sometimes, students don't recognise opportunities for learning unless someone explicitly tells them. It is important to recognise the potential of every encounter and situation to be a learning opportunity and you must seek out people, information and experiences that will enhance your learning. Add some ideas to your SWOT or SNOB table.

Consider the threats or barriers to your learning. Are these threats or barriers from the physical environment, the organisation of students' support, or are there internal barriers within yourself which hinder your learning? Add them to your SWOT or SNOB table.

There is no outline answer at the end of the chapter, as Table 2.5 provides an illustrative example of a completed SWOT analysis using information from Bobby's scenario within the various activities of this chapter.

Your SWOT or SNOB should look similar in construction to Table 2.5, but it will contain your own individual personal analysis of your strengths, weaknesses, needs, opportunities, threats, or barriers.

Strengths	Weaknesses
Professional skills: I am a good communicator (NMC competencies self-assessment, personal qualities self-assessment and mentor feedback). *Professional knowledge and skills:* I have good knowledge of medicines and accurate numeracy skills (NMC competencies, Skills clusters self-assessment and feedback from mentors). *Professional attitudinal values:* I have an inclusive attitude towards patients and colleagues (mentor feedback and professional colleagues' Johari window assessment). *Academic knowledge* I am a multi-modal learner, gaining experience from all four learning styles. I am particularly strong in the Read–Write category of the VARK questionnaire. *Personal strengths:* I am well organised and always seek support for assignments and practice learning. (Personal Self-efficacy self-assessment, feedback from university assignment tutors and reflection with personal tutor).	*Professional skills:* I need to involve myself more with the children's parents and family – promoting good parenting and explaining their role in home care (NMC competencies self-assessment and feedback from mentors). I need to develop my assertiveness to be involved in learning clinical skills (personal qualities self-assessment and mentor feedback). *Professional knowledge and attitudinal values:* I don't always understand patients' and families' specific religious needs (NMC competencies self-assessment, mentor feedback and significant event reflections). *Academic knowledge and skills:* I struggled to achieve a 2:1 grade in the first assignment of Year 3 to maintain my 2:1 classification (Exams and assessments feedback and Level 6 grading criteria).
Opportunities	**Threats**
My next practice placement has lots of opportunities for learning (Placement website information): Rotation through general care, out-patients and PICU. I have an allocated mentor with off-duty already planned. This is a well organised placement, so it is an opportunity for me to stay well organised too.	*Personal attitudinal values and skills:* My own self-efficacy is low when faced with high demands on my time from home, university and placement. *Personal and professional attitude* and organisational skills: I sometimes find some of the staff impatient, because I am not assertive enough to explain my learning needs (Personal qualities self-assessment).

Table 2.5 Example of a completed SWOT analysis, showing self-assessment tools used and evidence for findings

Activity 2.5 should have helped you to analyse all of your self-assessment findings in order to:

- recognise those elements where you are achieving, or exceeding, expectations;
- understand your weaknesses or needs;

- consider a wide range of learning opportunities;
- acknowledge perceived or actual barriers or threats to your learning.

Knowing yourself through this thorough self-assessment and SWOT or SNOB analysis will enable you to negotiate your access to learning opportunities. This will make the fundamental difference between steering your own transition journey through self-agency, or letting someone else determine it for you; potentially ending up with a less than satisfactory experience. Use your new self-understanding to, *Have the confidence to say to the staff on the ward that's what you want to do, or that's what you want to learn* (Grace, Child Branch student) (Major 2010, p207).

Having completed the SWOT or SNOB analysis, it is now time to draw the chapter to a close.

Chapter summary

This chapter has explained the principles, presented examples, and provided activities, for you to be able to:

- undertake and record your own personal, professional and academic self-assessments that are relevant to the transition from student to newly registered nurse;
- undertake a SWOT or SNOB analysis of all of your transition-focussed self-assessments in order to 'know yourself' in your current role, ready to make TFPDPs that will guide you towards achievement of the knowledge, skills and attitudes, mind-set and resilience expected of the newly registered nurse role.

You should now have a good idea of:

- your personal, professional and academic strengths – the things you want to *keep doing* to maintain your current standards and improvements;
- your personal, professional and academic weaknesses or learning needs, which you want to *start developing;*
- the barriers or threats to your learning which you want to *stop being a hindrance* and develop positively, while using every available opportunity to support your learning.

All of the self-assessment information gained through your SWOT or SNOB analysis should be considered to be constructive feedback and can now be used to 'feed-forward' into the construction of your own individualised TFPDPs. These can be used as a personal guide and shared with your mentors and academic tutors, to provide a strong sense of personal ownership and direction, open up learning opportunities and verify achievements during the transition journey. Personal Development Planning will be explored in depth in Chapter 3.

Activities: brief outline answers

Activity 2.1 Reflection (page 30)

Your consideration of Zanadi's reassessment of his abilities may include the sort of steps that you have seen patients go through when they have experienced a sudden life-changing illness. Steps of the grieving process are similar to the stages of transition: shock, denial, anger, resentment. With positive support, people undergoing dramatic change often find renewed energy and determination to disengage from their previous role and re-incorporate themselves into society in a new role. They often want to find out everything they can about their 'new way of life', pushing the limits of their boundaries in order to achieve new goals.

Activity 2.2 Critical thinking (page 32)

Bobby might have chosen the following self-assessments as having personal relevance:

Self-assessment	Personal, professional, or academic	Knowledge, skills, or attitudinal values	Reason for choice
NMC competencies. (See Professional Development record.)	Professional	K, S, AV	I have to pass these to register. I need to know what I currently can and can't do and work towards them.
Job description local children's ward.	Professional	K, S, AV	I want this job and must work towards the job's KSF requirements.
NHS Leadership Academy. Belbin team roles.	Professional	K, S and AV	This year I have to be able to lead the team for Registration competence and my new job. I want to see what type of team player I am.
Johari window (Luft) (ask friends to do).	Personal	AV	A good self-awareness tool for building self-esteem. (What they might say is a bit daunting, but will help me build public interpersonal relationships.)
Johari window (ask colleagues to do).	Professional	AV	Am I really doing as well as I think?
Personal qualities for learning inventory (Major). Personal self-efficacy scale (Chen, Gully and Eden). Learning styles inventory (Honey and Mumford), or Fleming and Mills' VARK. University level 6 grading criteria. Academic feedback.	Academic Professional Personal	K, S	I want a 2:1 degree classification and to pass competencies at first attempt. I need to be self-sufficient in my learning and need an awareness of how I currently learn best. Perhaps I could expand my personal qualities and learning styles to capitalise on learning opportunities now and throughout my career.

Table 2.6 Possible transition-focussed self-assessment tools and sources of evidence for your achievements

Activity 2.4 Reflection and critical thinking (page 41)

You will possibly be seeing the same abilities being apparent in several of the self-assessments: for example, several sources of evidence may be saying that you have good communication skills. Similarly, some of your weaknesses, or learning needs, will be duplicated. Having undertaken several self-assessments that endorse each other's findings will give you the reassurance of what your strengths and weaknesses, or learning needs, actually are. There may also be some strengths and weaknesses or needs that show up in one assessment but not in others – it is also important to record these.

Further reading

Akerjordet, K and Severinsson, E (2008) Emotionally intelligent nurse leadership: A literature review study. *Journal of Nursing Management*, 16: 565–77.

This article explains the usefulness of emotional intelligence for managing oneself in the role of nurse leadership.

Cowan, J (2010) Developing the ability for making evaluative judgements. Teaching in Higher Education, 15(3): 323–34. www.tandfonline.com/doi/abs/10.1080/13562510903560036

Contains practical ideas about how to develop the ability to make evaluative judgements.

Helms, MM and Nixon, J (2010) Exploring SWOT analysis – where are we now?: A review of academic research from the last decade. *Journal of Strategy and Management* 3(3): 215–51. http://dx.doi.org/10.1108/17554251011064837

A useful history of SWOT and SNOB analysis.

Nash, R, Lemcke, P and Sacre, S (2009) Enhancing transition: An enhanced model of clinical placement for final year nursing students. *Nurse Education Today*, 29(1): 48–56.

In this article, you can read about how student learning is organised to enhance learning in the final year. It may give you some ideas about what opportunities might exist in your own placements.

Ong, G-L (2013) Using final placements to prepare student nurses. *Nursing Times*, 109(3): 12–14.

This short article will also help you to consider what to learn and how you want to learn in final placement.

Pitt, V, Powis, D, Levett-Jones, T and Hunter, S (2014) The influence of personal qualities on performance and progression in a pre-registration nursing programme. *Nurse Education Today*, 34(5): 866–71. http://dx.doi.org/10.1016/j.nedt.2013.10.011

This recent research with student nurses explains more about how personal qualities can be understood to help plan learning experiences.

Useful websites

Further information about a variety of Emotional Intelligence testing tools and SWOT and SNOB analysis can be accessed at the following sites:

www.mindtools.com

www.eiconsortium.org/measures/weis.html

Chapter 3

Transition-focussed reflection and personal development planning

Joanne Keeling and Denise Major

NMC Standards for Pre-registration Nursing Education

This chapter will address the following competencies:

Domain 1: Professional values

Generic competencies:

5. All nurses must fully understand the nurse's various roles, responsibilities and functions, and adapt their practice to meet the changing needs of people, groups, communities and populations.

7. All nurses must be responsible and accountable for keeping their knowledge and skills up to date through continuing professional development. They must aim to improve their performance and enhance the safety and quality of care through evaluation, supervision and appraisal.

8. All nurses must practise independently, recognising the limits of their competence and knowledge. They must reflect on these limits and seek advice from, or refer to, other professionals where necessary.

Domain 2: Communication and interpersonal skills

Generic competencies:

3. All nurses must use the full range of communication methods, including verbal, non-verbal and written, to acquire, interpret and record their knowledge and understanding of people's needs. They must be aware of their own values and beliefs and the impact this may have on their communication with others. They must take account of the many different ways in which people communicate and how these may be influenced by ill health, disability and other factors, and be able to recognise and respond effectively when a person finds it hard to communicate.

(Continued)

(Continued)

Domain 3: Nursing practice and decision making

Generic competencies:

1. All nurses must use up-to-date knowledge and evidence to assess, plan, deliver and evaluate care, communicate findings, influence change and promote health and best practice. They must make person-centred, evidence-based judgments and decisions, in partnership with others involved in the care process, to ensure high quality care. They must be able to recognise when the complexity of clinical decisions requires specialist knowledge and expertise, and consult or refer accordingly.

Domain 4: Leadership, management and team working

Generic competencies:

4. All nurses must be self-aware and recognise how their own values, principles and assumptions may affect their practice. They must maintain their own personal and professional development, learning from experience, through supervision, feedback, reflection and evaluation.
5. All nurses must facilitate nursing students and others to develop their competence, using a range of professional and personal development skills.

Essential Skills Clusters

This chapter will address the following ESCs:

Cluster: Care, compassion and communication

1. As partners in the care process, people can trust a newly registered graduate nurse to provide collaborative care based on the highest standards, knowledge and competence.

First progression point:

1.2. Works within limitations of the role and recognises own level of competence.

Second progression point:

1.7. Uses professional support structures to learn from experience and make appropriate adjustments.

Entry to the register:

1.9.   Is self-aware and self-confident, knows own limitations and is able to take appropriate action.

1.14.   Uses professional support structures to develop self-awareness, challenge own prejudices and enable professional relationships, so that care is delivered without compromise.

Chapter aims

After reading this chapter, you will be able to:

- describe the purpose of reflection and explain its significance to your personal development as a nurse;
- appreciate the advantages and disadvantages of using a reflective model to examine and make sense of your own experiences;
- have an awareness of some strategies for critical thinking and focussing your reflection on your own development needs during the transition period;
- recognise the importance of self-assessment and personal development planning in the transition to registered nurse status and beyond;
- construct a TFPDP that will assist you in meeting your development needs and prepare you for professional practice.

Introduction

Scenario

Kendi is a third year nursing student who is about to begin the final placement of the nursing programme on a surgical ward. Kendi is looking forward to this placement and is very confident of being successful in achieving the final competencies of the nursing programme, in order to be eligible for entry onto the professional register. With confidence growing, from having experienced similar ward placements in the past, and always achieving the required competencies and positive reports from practice mentors, Kendi considers that achieving competence is well within reach. Kendi has personal confidence in performing nursing skills such as neurological observations, setting up infusions and calculating medication dosages.

(Continued)

(Continued)

However, from undertaking a quick self-assessment prior to this final placement, Kendi has decided that the main areas to strengthen are leadership and management skills, as there has been limited experience of delegation available until the previous placement in Year 3. Kendi considers that the third year of a nursing programme is all about management and leadership in preparation for taking charge as a registered nurse; thus, has written a personal development plan that focusses upon practising skills in delegation, with a smaller development plan for merely refining what Kendi considers to be already good communication skills. Kendi feels sure that, with minimal work, achievement of the final competencies are well within grasp and could be passed with flying colours as had been done in the past.

However, during the third week of placement an unplanned situation occurrs for. Kendi is asked by a mentor to sit, and spend some time with, the distressed partner of a man having surgery that day, in order to find out what her worries are and how she might be reassured. Kendi is at a loss, having not envisaged that preparing for qualification as a nurse would involve this type of care, always having thought that this might be the role of the healthcare assistants or chaplaincy service, as that was how it was done in previous placements. Kendi has experience with speaking to relatives and carers of patients, but mainly as an observer with a mentor taking the lead.

Kendi suddenly feels not as prepared for professional practice as first thought, feeling uncomfortable and not knowing what to say; and so asked the mentor if this care could be delegated to somebody else. Kendi's mentor is taken aback and asks Kendi to reflect on this response to the situation and to develop a personal development plan for discussion. Kendi is embarrassed and does not know where to start.

The scenario above highlights that no matter how prepared we think we may be, nursing practice sometimes throws us a curve ball. In the scenario above Kendi appears to have not taken the time to assess personal and professional progress thoroughly and may have manipulated previous personal development plans to address what Kendi believed being a third year student nurse was about. In short Kendi appears not to have seen the bigger picture.

As you will have read in previous chapters, the stages of transition from student to registered nurse can be a stressful and busy time and to manage this it is perhaps easier to focus on proficiency in nursing tasks and physical clinical skills than it is to consider the wider scope of nursing practice. Perhaps Kendi managed stress by avoiding reflecting on the skills and attitudinal values required during patient interaction, in order to have what Kendi thought may have been an easier transition. However, it is very important that as a registered nurse we are able to think critically and this should begin by thinking critically about *ourselves* which may at times be uncomfortable.

This chapter discusses the concept of critical thinking through reflection and reflective practice, with particular emphasis on transition-focussed reflection. Some definitions of reflection and its significance to your personal development as a nurse will be explored. We will consider reflective models and encourage you to appreciate the advantages and disadvantages of using a reflective model to examine and make sense of your own experiences. This will help you to think critically and to make choices about the tools you use to assist you to manage your own development. Finally, we will look at some practical advice in terms of personal development planning and consider how you can build a personal development plan in preparation for professional practice and beyond.

What is reflection?

You may be familiar with the term 'reflection' and have had the opportunity to engage in 'reflective writing' as part of your nursing studies. The ability of a student nurse to reflect, and evidence this process, is made explicit in Domain 4, Generic competence 4, as above (NMC, 2010). There are various theories about reflection, which are presented in the following concept summary.

Concept summary: Reflection

John Dewey (1859–1952), the American philosopher, psychologist and educational reformer, is acknowledged as being instrumental in the development of the concept of reflection through his early works. For Dewey, reflection was a process of inquiry in which the learner applied critical thought to a situation in an attempt to learn and apply this new learning in the future. Reflection for him was purposeful and was

> *active, persistent and careful consideration of any belief or supposed form of knowledge in the light of the grounds that support it, and further conclusions to which it leads ... it includes a conscious and voluntary effort to establish belief upon a firm basis of evidence and rationality.*

(Dewey, 1933, p9)

Dewey was a pragmatist and saw reflection as a vehicle for *learning in order to 'think well'*; in short he saw reflection as a purposeful tool for developing critical thinking in order to develop oneself and to avoid repetitive and routine action and simple assimilation of knowledge. Dewey's criteria of the concept of reflection were as follows:

1. Reflection is concerned with making sense of a situation in order to enable the learner to transfer this understanding to other experiences in the future in order to personally develop.

(Continued)

(Continued)

2. Reflection is a different way of thinking and requires systematic 'unpicking of issues' in a scientific like way.

3. Reflection cannot be a solely individual exercise and needs to occur with feedback and interaction with others in order to test out perceptions and ideas.

4. The attitude and values of the learner are important in order for reflection to take place: a commitment to personal development is essential.

(Rodgers, 2002)

For Dewey reflection was concerned with using experience as a means by which to continually move forward and to develop thinking and personal theory. In short, reflection is concerned with continual personal development. Dewey's work is still widely cited today and remains seminal in terms of its importance to education practice and theory. Dewey's work has later been developed by a number of authors who have built on Dewey's original theory of reflection in order to apply it to different practice educational settings such as music (Bauer and Dunn, 2003) and art education (Goldblatt, 2006).

Reflection as a concept inherent within the teaching and learning approach has been increasingly present in nursing education since the 1980s and has been widely influenced by the work of Donald Schön (1983;1987). Schön was concerned with how reflection is relevant to practice and organisational settings. He spoke of 'organisational learning' (p254) and was interested in how individuals learned from personal experience as opposed to pure knowledge acquisition. Schön proposed reflection as a form of action and situated it within professional contexts. He proposed two types of reflection in practice – reflection 'on action' and reflection 'in action'. Schön proposed that the novice practitioner reflects on action and looks back at a situation after the event in order to analyse it and develop further action. Reflection in action was attributed to the more experienced practitioner, who can reflect while in the event or situation and adjust their actions as a result of being able to process and problem solve while the event is occurring in real time.

This theory complements the work of a contemporary of Schön, Patricia Benner, the nursing theorist and academic. Benner's work 'From novice to expert' (1982) was a result of her acknowledgement that nursing practice was an evolving discipline in which it was no longer adequate that nurses should be guided by instruction and routine practice. Benner spoke of nurses as needing to be critical thinkers increasingly reliant upon their own experiential learning and interpretation of novel events. Benner's concept of the 'novice to expert' nurse is reliant on the importance of situational learning and thus the knowledge that is derived from the nurses' experience of situations. Similar to Dewey and Schön, she posits that reflective practice and the ability to reflect are essential for the personal and skills development of the nurse.

Later, Mezirow (1991) explained reflection as transforming meaning into learning. He described a process by which adult learners made sense of experiences and therefore came to an interpretation of their experiences on which they could base future actions and decisions. In this way Mezirow termed meaning as becoming learning and this theory he called 'transformative learning': a process of effecting change in practice as the result of deriving meaning from experience. The significance of Mezirow's work to nursing education is that he stated the link between theory and practice and saw transformative learning as the route to critical thinking. As nursing is a profession that involves the ability to think critically in practice situations, it is no surprise that his work remains important in nursing education today.

Before we go on to look at what tools might help you to reflect on your practice, please complete the activity below which will give you a starting point for reflection. This quote from Huxley (cited in Kegan, 1983, p11) may help you to complete the activity: *Experience is not what happens to you, it's what you do with what happens to you.*

Activity 3.1   Critical thinking

Think about a situation that you have encountered recently that made you think, whether this be a situation in practice, at home, alone or with friends. Take some time to describe the situation: what happened? where did it happen? who was involved? when did it happen? This is the situation.

Now think about *your experience* of this situation; what did you feel and experience as a result of the situation at the time. What have you since thought about it in terms of your own thoughts and feelings and what have you done or thought about doing as a result? This is your experience of the situation and will form the basis of your reflection.

As this answer is based on your own observation, there is no outline answer at the end of the chapter.

Why is reflection significant to your personal development as a nurse?

In reference to our values and attitudes, as nurses we abide by a set of professional values set out in The Code (NMC, 2015). We are also required to meet certain standards as a registered nurse set out in the standards for competence for registered nurses (NMC, 2010). However, not only are we expected to meet the standards, we are also expected to maintain them throughout our careers and show evidence of this through our practice, our attitude and behaviour and through the NMC's revalidation process. As part of the nurses' revalidation requirements we are required to show our ability to reflect both by completing reflective accounts and engaging in a reflective discussion with another nurse registrant.

In the period of transition from a student nurse to a registered nurse it is useful to have an understanding of the standards for competence for registered nurses and how you will seek to achieve these in order to enter and remain on the professional register. You will have read previously in Chapter 1 about the increased responsibility that you will encounter as a registered nurse, and will have learned about some strategies that may help you to deal with this during your transition period. The ability to reflect and make use of your experiences in order to learn and adapt your approach and actions, will be an important strategy for you to practise and refine, not only through the transition period but throughout your nursing career.

If we look back at Dewey's theory, it appears to sit well within the profession of nursing in that as nurses we are required to think critically in complex situations and propose or change our actions as a result, that is, to take a pragmatic approach. This was the basis of Benner's work in the 1980s in that she recognised the changing nature of acute and complex nursing care and understood that nurses would be required to think while 'doing' and be able to problem solve using personal experience, rather than relying on traditional practice and reference to academic text. Nursing in the modern era requires a nurse to be able to solve complex problems and to care for patients holistically. In order to do this and care for our patients we must value nursing knowledge of the past, but we must also be prepared to contribute to that knowledge through experiential learning that can translate to evidence based practice for the next generation of nurses. In short, through being reflective thinkers we are better placed to ensure that nursing is visible (Weir-Hughes, 2016) and of prime benefit to the patients in ever-increasing multi-professional models of care.

As nurses, we are constantly working with others, whether this be multidisciplinary and inter-professionally or within nursing teams. As such, as a registered nurse you should have the opportunity to liaise with and reflect on issues with others through formal mechanisms such as clinical supervision, appraisal, preceptorship and Schwartz rounds (Pepper *et al.*, 2012). This means that through the very nature of the nursing role, you will be in the privileged position to be able to invite others to feed back to you on your thoughts, ideas and performance and use this as part of improving your practice.

Models of reflection

We have considered some of the theory and definitions of reflection and the purpose of reflection to your personal development as a nurse. We will now consider reflective models and how they might help you to structure your thoughts on your experiences in order to reflect and learn to effect change. A reflective model can be used as a way to organise and thoroughly consider your thoughts, feelings and subsequent action planning following experiencing a situation. A reflective model uses cue questions or phrases in an attempt to guide you through the process of reflecting on a situation. The purpose of a reflective model is to enable you to extract the meaning and hence learning from your observations, thoughts and feelings. In this respect, you are able to develop new insights and meanings that will enable you to consider alternative or new actions for the future. While there are many reflective models, they all follow a similar cycle in that they prompt the reflector to travel from one position to considering other alternatives and to arrive at an action plan. While there are numerous reflective models we will consider three of the most widely used models of reflection in nursing education; the first being that of Gibbs (1988).

As you can see from Figure 3.1, Gibbs guides the reflector through the reflective cycle starting with a description of an event. Next he directs the reflector to consider your thinking and feelings about that event. Remember Activity 3.1 and your consideration of your thoughts and feelings about a situation and how this differed from the initial description of the event. You will see that you have more than likely addressed the first two cue stages of Gibbs' cycle.

The next stage of Gibbs' cycle is the evaluation stage and is useful in prompting the reflector to look at both the positive and negative aspects of the experience. This is important as often a student nurse will focus on the negative aspects of a situation as opposed to the positive aspects. This may be due to a lack of self-confidence and a desire to 'fix' perceived gaps in knowledge or skill, especially during the time of transition from student nurse to registrant. However, it is important to celebrate the positive

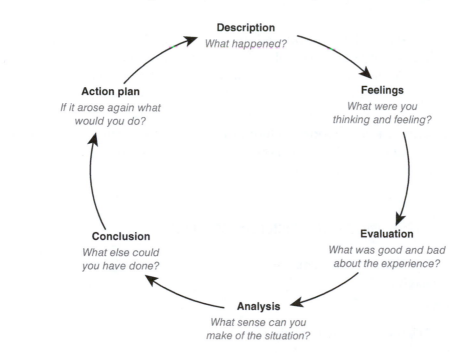

Figure 3.1 Gibbs' reflective cycle 1988

aspects of the situation and to consider any negative perceptions as opportunities for learning and development.

The analysis stage of Gibbs' reflective cycle directs the reflector to try to make sense of the situation. It is here that you may wish to consider your own previous experiences and knowledge and to do some further research as to whether the key points that you have raised are addressed in academic literature and discourse. The analysis stage enables you to thoroughly consider what your understanding is of the situation, what explanations may exist and what this means for you and your practice.

The conclusion stage enables you to summarise the outcome of your thinking and from your experience and your research to consider different ways in which you may approach the situation in the future. Any action planning as a result of this needs to be focussed on your development and enables you to test out new courses of actions should a similar issue arise in the future.

Activity 3.2 Reflection

Consider the situation you used to think about in Activity 3.1. Now apply Gibbs' reflective cycle to structure your thoughts about this situation. Consider each stage of the cycle in turn and ensure that you focus each stage on yourself and what you would like to explore in terms of further learning.

As this answer is based on your own observation, there is no outline answer at the end of the chapter.

Another widely used model in nursing education is that of Johns (1995). Johns' model on first glance looks a little more complex than that of Gibbs but is comprehensive in that it guides the reflector through different aspects of learning. Johns' model incorporated and was based on the work of Carper (1978) who wrote of 'fundamental patterns of knowing in nursing'. The patterns of knowing in nursing were empirical, personal, ethical and aesthetic. Johns' model includes these ways of knowing but he includes reflexivity as a way of connecting reflection to past experiences. Below is an outline of Johns' Model of Structured Reflection:

Johns' (1995) Model of structured reflection

Write a description of the experience.
Cue questions:

- Aesthetics
    o What was I trying to achieve?
    o Why did I respond as I did?

- o   What were the consequences of that for the patient, to others and myself?
- o   How was this person feeling (Or these persons)?
- o   How did I know this?

- • Personal:
  - o   How did I feel in this situation?
  - o   What internal factors were influencing me?

- • Ethics:
  - o   How did my actions match with my beliefs?
  - o   What factors made me act in incongruent ways?

- • Empirics:
  - o   What knowledge did or should have informed me?

- • Reflexivity:
  - o   How does this connect with previous experiences?
  - o   Could I handle this better in similar situations?
  - o   What would be the consequences of alternative actions for the patient, others and myself?
  - o   How do I now feel about this experience?
  - o   Can I support myself and others better as a consequence?
  - o   Has this changed my ways of knowing?

You may wish to complete Activity 3.2 using Johns' (1995) model in order to compare and contrast using this model with that of Gibbs.

An alternative reflective model that you may wish to consider, to assist your thinking through a situation, is John Driscoll's reflective cycle (1994). Driscoll's model is based upon three key questions from the work of American teacher Terry Borton (1970):

1.   What?

2.   So What?

3.   Now What?

Driscoll links these key questions to experience and offers cue questions to enable the reflector to think through a situation from different perspectives focussing on the 'What? So What? And Now What?' Driscoll's model may be easy to remember and apply at face value, being composed of only three components. However, it is important to remember the cue questions that Driscoll proposes to ensure that a thorough reflective process is engaged. Hence for the novice reflector Driscoll's model may not provide enough overt structure and could easily be misused as a quick fix option for reflection. This would lead to a reflective process that lacks depth and focus on self which is the antithesis of the purpose of reflection: the aim of reflection being to focus the reflector on self-development and enable examination of new knowledge or synthesis.

We have looked here at three reflective models but there are many more to investigate. It is important that you read about reflective models and consider a number in order to select the one that you feel would best help you to organise your thoughts and feelings into a coherent baseline for identifying your development needs. This is especially important during the time of transition as you will have read that this can be a time of increased anxiety and doubt, in terms of your own skills and knowledge and readiness for professional practice as a registrant. As such it would be easy to identify countless development needs without a basis in any evidence. A reflective model can be used as a tool for gathering the evidence for development based on your experiences, and so can help you to plan a more transition-focussed plan.

Why use a reflective model?

There has been much academic debate in the literature about the use of reflective models and whether we should be using these as a way to assess and develop student nurses' reflective skills. Some authors argue that using reflective models to assess student nurses' leads to a mechanical and restrictive approach that has the opposite effect of that which we would encourage. Coward (2011) has observed that students may find the use of a reflective model a chore that needs performing in order to pass an assessed task. She also expresses concerns about the honesty and ability of student nurses to engage in truthful reflection if they may be worried about professional judgement in terms of things they may have experienced which may be unprofessional or at odds with The Code (NMC, 2015). She therefore advocates using narratives and humour as points of reflection and as teaching methods, in which the true story may be explored by the student without fear of failed assessment or professional judgement. Narrative or story telling has also been explored in other fields such as psychology and is now a popular methodology within contemporary research to explore people's lived experience of an issue or event. Hence the value of using scenarios to learn from events.

Indeed, there are many ways in which we may encourage reflection and that you may wish to explore as an alternative to structured models. Chan (2014) explored poetry writing as an alternative to reflective writing in that by its very nature of being an expressive form it is more akin to exploring inner feelings. Coleman and Willis (2015) studied student nurses' perceptions of poetry writing and concluded that poetry writing as a form of reflection could prompt freedom of self-expression and provide students with a sense of self-satisfaction.

However you choose to reflect on your practice, using the higher order skills of reflection and reflexivity will ultimately enable you to create good quality, well informed personal development plans (Quality Assurance Agency for Higher Education (QAA), 2007), which will help you to meet your professional obligation to recognise and address deficits in your knowledge and skills (NMC, 2010). In Kendi's example, the insight gained from reflective discussion with the mentor prompted consideration of the need to be more aware of the NMC competencies for registration. Becoming aware of one short-coming should have prompted Kendi to seek out whether there were also other short-comings in preparation for the registered nurse role. The use of a reflective model can assist in providing an awareness of growth in attitudes, as well as knowledge and skills.

Kendi may wish to reflect again on the attitude used in supporting relatives and the general attitudinal values exhibited towards professional interpersonal relationships. Using Johns' model, Kendi could have recognised that the internal factors of not knowing the professional obligations to the NMC competencies had produced incongruent actions and undesirable consequences for self, colleagues, the patient and their family. Kendi may have recognised the need for better self-support by actually knowing how to perform against the NMC competencies.

In exploring the issues that arise from using a reflective model, supportive reading is required in order to undertake the analysis posed by the cue questions of the model. The analysis might include using relevant self-assessment tools to generate an overall picture of strengths, weaknesses or learning needs, opportunities to learn, and threats or barriers to learning, as discussed in Chapter 2.

Kendi could have used the NMC competency statements as a self-assessment tool to provide heightened awareness of knowledge, skills and attitudes in relation to *all* of the competencies, not just the communication aspect that the mentor had highlighted.

The final part of the reflective models asks the reader to consider how they could plan to overcome whatever the issues were that you identified, or what they could do differently next time, or 'now what' is to be done to further their learning or abilities?

Gibbs' model describes this as the 'action planning' phase. The other two models also show similarities in their need for action to cope differently with the situation next time it occurs.

The action planning phase of a reflective model could also be termed 'personal development planning', which is driven by a comprehensive self-assessment as the first stage. As stated above, this comes either from the model cues themselves, or from further self-assessments that the findings might prompt.

When used within a supportive learning environment, action plans, or personal development plans, can communicate learning needs and goals, provide strong motivation for learning and progressively create a sense of personally grounded achievement and self-confidence. This achievement and self-confidence is particularly enhanced when reflection and reflexivity are used again to evaluate progress within the final point of the plan (QAA, 2007; Major, 2015). Transition-focussed personal development planning will be explored in the next section of this chapter.

Personal development planning

Introduction

Following on from the reflections on practice in the earlier part of this chapter and the self-assessment examples of Chapter 2, the next part of this chapter will provide guidance so that you can use your own SWOT or SNOB analysis to create your own, individually tailored TFPDP (Major, 2015). Your TFPDP will serve as a supportive guide, learning agreement and record of achievement as you complete your student journey towards registration as a professional nurse. The process of personal development planning needs to be driven by you, yourself, in a proactive manner, so as to drive your own career positively.

Concept summary: personal development planning

What is a Personal Development Plan (PDP) used for?

- A PDP can be used for professional career planning and for personal guidance.
- A PDP serves as a guide for self-development and evaluation of your achievements.
- A PDP is your articulation of your intended learning for your professional career; it can incorporate professional, academic and personal goals to help you to achieve your professional development. Fulfilling students' own particular learning needs builds students' competence, confidence and satisfaction (Major, 2010).

Who uses PDP?

- Anyone can use a PDP. The Dearing Report (Dearing, 1997) recommended their introduction as an outcome of work on progress files for Higher Education (HE) students. Dearing (1997) saw them as a supportive measure to provide transparent personal development plans for all HE students, to demonstrate their fitness for employment into their specific chosen career (QAA, 2007).
- They are personal to the person writing them.
- They are for yourself, to communicate your learning needs and intended learning resources, actions and strategies to yourself and your learning facilitators.
- Each person's PDP will be unique to them.

When should you use a PDP?

- whenever you need one;
- for whatever purpose you need it;
- to organise your thoughts, to relieve stress and prevent panic;
- personally – to organise your personal life and home demands in relation to your professional career;
- professionally – to drive your career or meet registration and employment targets;
- academically – to plan work and achieve academic awards.

Why should you use a PDP?

- It can serve as a 'learning agreement' – a sort of 'contract' between you and your learning facilitators so that each appreciates and agrees their part in the learning development process.
- You can be your own facilitator.
- Someone else may be helping to facilitate your learning and development and need to know your needs: mentor, supervisor in practice, and academic tutors.
- Personal development planning, as a strategy for your own lifelong professional development, will help you to identify needs and set goals, so that, as you approach and embark upon your career as a qualified nurse, you have some idea of your pathway for the future (Burton and Ormrod, 2011).

Where should you store your PDP?

- in your personal Professional Development Record (PDR), or in your Professional Portfolio; in your professional career as a registered nurse, a personal development plan could be a part of your professional preceptorship plan, or a part of your annual appraisal.

How should you construct your PDP?

- issues arising from the self-assessments;
- SMART learning objectives;
- resources, actions and strategies;
- evidence of achievement;
- review date;
- results of review.

This is a standard, sequential format that provides an easily recognisable style, has logical progression and should have space for endorsement signatures. There are commercial examples of PDPs available, but you can also self-generate. They all have the same basic structure and style.

You may be familiar with the template suggested within the personal development planning documentation provided by your own university. This chapter will use the template in Figure 3.2, as its headings are clear and unambiguous.

Name:

Personal Development Plan in relation to:

Self-assessment and Date	Learning objectives	Resources Actions and Strategies	Success criteria (Evidence of achievement)	Review date	Results of review (Evaluation of progress)

Signature of Student ....Date...........................

Signature of Practice Mentor ....Date...........................

Signature of Personal Tutor/Academic supervisor..Date...........................

Figure 3.2   Example Personal Development Plan template

We will now begin to construct the content of your TFPDP.

Activity 3.3   Communicating the purpose of a PDP

Print off, or construct your own electronic or paper copy of the PDP template.
If you are going to use a paper copy, have a pencil and eraser to hand so that you can easily alter it as your thoughts develop. Remember to ink it in before it is shared with your personal tutor or mentor. Better still, use an electronic template, so that you can easily cut and paste to move or alter content.

Fill in your name. Now add the title and the overall goal of your personal development plan, for example: 'Transition-Focussed Personal Development Plan: Year 3 to achieve Nursing & Midwifery Council Registration as RN (Adult /Children & Young People/Mental Health)'

As this activity is personal to you, there is no outline answer at the end of the chapter.

The development plan is now personalised to you and your current transition journey. Of course, this template can be used for any personal development planning, but for the purpose of this chapter, the content will be customised to reflect your transition-focused self-assessment analysis.

Figure 3.3 provides some cues as to how to construct each column in the systematic way from the top down and from left to right to follow the process of assessment, planning for implementation and evaluating. The assessment is a summary of the learning needs identified from all of your critical reflections and self-assessments that emerged from your SWOT or SNOB analysis. Planning is the setting of specific, measurable, achievable, realistic, time-related (SMART) learning objectives (Doran, 1981) along with planning what resources you will use and the actions and strategies that you will employ to use the resources. You must also plan for what will constitute evidence of achievement of your learning objectives. After implementation, the evidence of achievement can be reviewed so as to form the evaluation of your learning progress. The results of the review cannot be written into the plan until you have undertaken your learning, or reached the review date.

Having looked at the blank template, we now need to consider the actual words that we should use to convey accurate messages about our desired learning.

The TFPDP in Figure 3.4 provides an example of the actual words which you might use within your own TFPDP. This is only a brief example from one self-assessment for *professional* learning. The objectives contain action verbs from the affective domain of Bloom's (1956) taxonomy that will help you to recognise their achievement. The end-point review has not yet been undertaken.

You may devise shorter expressive ways of writing your PDPs from your SWOT or SNOB analysis, as there may be several self-assessments that lead you to the same learning need. You should write TFPDPs for academic, professional and personal issues.

The following discussion will guide you through the sequential construction of your TFPDP.

Assessment: using self-assessment analysis to identify learning needs

What issues to address?

- *personal* issues that impinge on your professional or academic work;
- *professional* development needs towards competence for registration:
    - practice assessment outcomes or programme requirements;
    - personal learning needs;
    - job role requirements in readiness for interview;
- *academic* assessment requirements.

Name:

Personal Development Plan in relation to:

Self-Assessment and Date	"SMART" Learning objectives (Doran, 1981)	Resources Actions and Strategies	Success Criteria (Evidence of achievement)	Review Date	Results of Review (Evaluation of Progress at review date) (Major, 2015, Adapted from Borton, 1970, p89).
DATE …	By (*time*) I will be able to (*verbs at correct levels from correct taxonomies*)	Plan of how I will meet the learning objectives	Written evidence	Matches the **Time** relation in the goal	"**What**" did I achieve for each of the learning objectives: Looking at my evidence of achievement, did I completely achieve the objective at the standard of performance set, partially achieve it or not achieve it at all; and why?
What have I assessed myself against?	in accordance with (*standard of performance*)	Resources to use	Endorsements from learning facilitator		
What are the issues from SWOT/SNOB analysis			Cross reference to other documents		"**So what**" importance does this have for me and my career: What have I learned about myself? Do I need to use a structured reflective model to make sense of the situation?
In relation to the issues:	Specific to the issue	Actions to take			
I can	Measurable by the verbs used	Strategies to use			
I can't					"**Now what**" can I do with this new knowledge, skill or attitude: How can it be used in my future work?
I need to	Achievable because it is a curriculum expectation of a learner at your level				How does this enhance my professional work?
Or					What benefits will this have for my patients? If I have not achieved the objective, can I carry over anything not completed to the next review date or make a new review date?
What do I know?	Realistic in time and level of learning and in the expectations of the available learning experiences				
What can I do?					
How do I feel?					
What don't I know?					
What can't I do?	Time related				
How should I feel?	1 week				
	1 month				
Or					
What do I want to know?	3 months				
What do I want to be able to do?	6 months				
How do I want to feel?	12 months				

Signature of Student .... Date...............

Signature of Practice Mentor .... Date...............

Signature of Personal Tutor/Academic supervisor .... Date...............

Figure 3.3 Example PDP construction

Source: Major (2015). Including adaptation of Borton's (1970, p89) 'reflective sequence' of 'What, So what, Now what'; with kind permission from McGraw Hill.

Name:

Transition-Focussed Personal Professional Development Plan: Year 3 'To achieve Nursing and Midwifery Council Registration as RN (Adult /Children and Young People / Mental Health)'

Self-Assessment and Date	Learning Objectives	Resources Actions and Strategies	Success Criteria (Evidence of achievement)	Review Date	Results of Review (Evaluation of Progress)
Date:				Mid-point semester 7	**What did I achieve?**
Having assessed myself against NMC (2010) competency Field standard 2,	1. During placement seven, I will **listen** to patients' views and **challenge** poor health behaviours.	Discuss my learning needs with my mentor. Ask for opportunities to work with patients/ clients who require health promotion.	I will have assisted one patient to make one positive change to their lifestyle which will promote their health.	Date:	I did not completely achieve this objective by midpoint, because I was working on other objectives. I have learned to listen to patients' views and to direct my own learning by being more assertive.
I need to develop my attitude positively towards those patients who have illness related to unhealthy lifestyle choices, by 'respecting people's rights to individual lifestyle choices while trying to promote health and education whenever possible.'	2. By the end of placement seven, I will **Participate actively** in promoting their health **and influence change**, while **justifying** the advice given, according to the requirements of competency field standard 2.	Read literature about health promotion methods and strategies. Use my therapeutic interpersonal skills to put these strategies in place.	I will write a structured reflection using Johns' (1995) model to demonstrate the effect of my behaviours which I have listed in the objective.		**So what importance does this have for me?** I must attend to this objective during the remainder of my placement in order to achieve competence for registration. **Now what can I do with this new knowledge, skill or attitude?** Continue actively listening to patient's views. Ask mentor to ensure suitable patient care experiences for this objective.
				End point review	*Write midpoint reviews for all of the other objectives.*
				Date:	*Write your review when you achieve an objective or reach the end point review date*

Signature of Student .... Date................

Signature of Practice Mentor .... Date................

Signature of Personal Tutor/Academic supervisor... Date................

Figure 3.4 Example of a completed TFPDP for one professional learning objective

Reflective assessment as described previously in Kendi's situation, using a model to reflect on professional practice, should be included, and may form the catalyst for deeper self-assessment against relevant documents, such as those discussed in Chapter 2, which tell you what you should be able to do by the time you reach registration.

Activity 3.4   Communicating your learning needs

It is important that you can write down your learning needs into your TFPDP so as to communicate them to your mentors in practice and to your academic tutors. Have another look at your work with Kendi earlier in the chapter and the activities with Bobby in Chapter 2, as all of the self-assessment tools that we explored there are relevant to you in some way or another. If you have not yet undertaken any reflections or self-assessments, now is the time to do them. You should then be able to summarise the findings from your reflections and self-assessments by making your SWOT or SNOB analysis. This summary should identify your learning needs, which can then be inserted into the self-assessment column of your TFPDP.

Although your SWOT/SNOB analysis and your learning needs will be individual to you, if you need some prompting, have another look at Bobby's SWOT analysis in Table 2.5 of Chapter 2.

Following on from the identification of learning needs, you can now set learning objectives to achieve them.

Planning: writing SMART learning objectives

You may have heard the terms goals, learning objectives and learning outcomes used interchangeably. Goals are generally the overall outcome desired, such as your goal 'To achieve Nursing & Midwifery Council Registration as RN (Adult/Children & Young People/Mental Health)' written into the title of your TFPDP. In order to achieve that goal, you will have found from your self-assessments that you have learning needs – thus you can set yourself learning outcomes or learning objectives to achieve these learning needs, which will ultimately achieve the goal of registration. Hence, for the purpose of writing your TFPDPs the second column should be headed 'Learning outcomes' or 'Learning objectives'. For ease of continuity, this chapter and Chapter 2, uses the term 'Learning objectives'.

Activity 3.5   Critical thinking – setting SMART learning objectives for the TFPDP

Select one of your learning needs and try to construct a SMART learning outcome based on the following information:

- be *specific*: setting individual learning objectives for each learning need makes them easily manageable and achievable. You have identified your learning needs in the first column of your TFPDP, now you need to set one or more learning objectives in order to meet each learning need. Only include one learning need within one learning objective;
- make the objective *measurable*: there is some debate about using behavioural objectives, but their strength lies in the fact that they describe observable *behaviours* – things that you and your assessors can see or hear you do that verify your achievements of your learning objectives. The measurable part of a learning objective sets the standard, or level, of performance required. Therefore, the taxonomies of learning can be useful tools for setting measurable objectives in all three domains;
- look again at Bloom's, Dave's and Harrow and Simpson's taxonomies of educational objectives – you could access these from the useful websites list at the end of the chapter;
- set your objectives using verbs or descriptive statements from all three domains of the educational taxonomy: cognitive, psychomotor and affective;
- make the objective *achievable and realistic*: select the appropriate level of learning that you wish to achieve, considering what level you are at now in any particular competence from your self-assessments and where you need to be by the end of your transition. Remember that it is acceptable to set incremental, stepped objectives over several weeks or months in order to reach the ultimate goal of competence in each domain. Setting small, achievable targets that together build towards the final goal will help you to gain confidence. Rather than constantly feeling that your overall goal is still a long way from reach, you will notice tangible progress;
- make the objective *time related*: each of your learning objectives needs a time boundary. This must also be realistic. For example, if your third year is split into three semesters and you need to achieve a certain level of competence by the middle of the final semester, then set your objectives for that learning need with lower levels of competence along the way as incremental, achievable, confidence-building steps for semesters one and two so that they lead you to that level of competence by the assessment date in semester 3. See the example in Figure 3.4. You might also wish to look at the useful websites list at the end of the chapter. When you are satisfied with the expression and meaning of your first learning objective, try writing learning objectives for the remainder of your identified learning needs and add them into your TFPDP.

(Continued)

(Continued)

You might find it helpful to discuss the writing of your learning objectives with your academic supervisor or personal tutor, or your mentor in practice.

Your individual learning objectives will be specific to you; however, Figure 3.4 should provide some ideas and there is a further explanation in the outline answer at the end of the chapter.

Having set your learning objectives in Activity 3.5, the next stage is planning how you will achieve these.

Planning: selecting and defining resources, actions and strategies

- A *resource* is something that aids your learning – mentors, clinical specialists, books, journals, reports, policies, standards for practice, real clinical equipment, models.
- An *action*, or *strategy*, is doing something with the resource – reading, watching/ observing, asking questions, practising under supervision. Using your own personal qualities to help manage your own learning; for example, being assertive, or communicating your needs.

The next planning column of the TFPDP asks you to consider the resources, actions and strategies that you will use to help you to achieve the learning objectives. Students often recognise learning strategies and resources that work well for them individually, but we can all benefit from sharing our ideas with others. Within Major's (2010) study, students identified several learning experiences that were very important to them during final placement, in order to achieve their specific learning needs for registration. There were also some situations that students found very unhelpful, so being assertive is a very important personal quality in order to keep the purpose of your learning clear to those who are supporting you. This should help to focus your placement experiences on undertaking learning activities that are aimed specifically towards achieving your learning objectives.

You might like to have a look at some of the findings from this study in Figure 3.5.

Good learning facilitation comes with a mentor who advocates for you, in order to 'open doors' to learning situations, who knows what you need and looks out for those opportunities through allocating you to specific patient care, or recommends you to someone else for you to go to a spoke placement or short learning experience such as

Final placement learning experiences identified by students as 'very important' from the quantitative findings	
Managing care	**Learning resources and strategies**
Managing the ward under supervision	Directing my own learning
Being given responsibility for a group of patients	Being able to access up to date resources for learning
Team work	Experiencing evidence-based practice
Being encouraged to participate in decisions about care	Being actively involved in the administration of medicines
Working alongside my mentor	Providing holistic care (total patient care) for patients under supervision
Attending MDT meetings	Talking with parents, carers or relatives of child/adult/ mental health patients/clients
Teaching	
Teaching students, parents, patients	Attending trained staff mandatory lectures and professional development sessions
Final placement learning experiences identified by students as 'very important' from the qualitative findings	
Positive learning environment	**Learning influenced by placement specialty**
Welcomed	Positive influence of placement specialty
Good communication	Learning specific care and conditions
Positive mentor attitude to teaching and learning	***Community learning opportunities***
Prior discussion of needs	Community nursing skills
Good resources, staff as a resource	Involvement/ independence in decision-making
Good teamwork	Caseload management
Good teaching	Visiting on my own pushed me to take the lead
Learning is seen as important	Confidence relating to patients
Learning opportunities	Wide range of cultural and religious needs
Variety of patients	Learning care from patient perspective
Variety of skills needed	Working with CPN
Could ask staff anything	Managing crisis
The assessment process helped learning	**Negative influence of placement specialty (barriers to learning)**
Transition learning opportunities	Too stressful, too busy to teach and learn
Rehearse first post	Too complex as many specialties on one ward
Have own workload	Pace too fast to explain complex drugs
More responsibility	Can't have own caseload

(Continued)

Figure 3.5   (Continued)

Less supervision	All decisions made by RNs
Supernumerary	**Expectations of final placement**
Working alongside mentor / mentoring team	Transfer from feeling like a student to feeling like a staff nurse
Appropriate staff expectations	Expectations from staff of performing a 'nearly qualified role'
Low student numbers rather than high student numbers	Supernumerary to focus on my needs not those of the service
Freedom in the team (independence)	Exceeded expectations … When staff helped prepare for interviews
Negative learning experiences	**Who helps with learning**
Not using my skills	Mentor, ward manager, other registered nursing staff
Lack of time with mentor	Self
Insufficient supervision	***How they help***
Too stressful to learn	Called me by my name
Long stay repetitive skills	Asked my needs
No flexible working	Asked what I wanted to join in with
Didn't feel part of the team	Included me (in the team)
Staff ignored me	Allocated appropriate caring
'You're just a student'	Were approachable
Given menial tasks / HCA/CSW work	Gave me responsibility
Not introducing themselves or me to others	Emotional support
The direct way staff speak to others	Shared experiences
Staff being stuck in their ways	Specialist skills
They expected too much from me – 'oh good, we've got a third year!'	Used my personal qualities – assertiveness, managing own learning, communication

Figure 3.5   Major, 2010, pp196–8, Table 15 (abridged)

an in-house lecture. It might be that the mentor takes you with them to shadow while they undertake some care or education of their own. However, for the mentor to know what you need on an individual level, it requires personal qualities of your own, such as good communication skills and resourcefulness to let your mentor know what you want to, and need to, learn, and how you would prefer to learn it.

Communication is not just verbal, based on what you see on the spur of the moment when you arrive at placement. Although having a mind-set to seize the opportunity for situational learning by linking conceptual and procedural knowledge is important, good communication of learning needs also requires forethought and planning so that your ideas are written down and rehearsed in your mind before you encounter the placements and classroom experiences.

A PDP is a three way 'contract' of learning between you, your personal teacher and your mentor, so that you can benefit from your own personal creation of ideas, express them clearly to others and benefit from the expertise and knowledge of your personal tutor and mentors. Your role in this is to prepare in advance by writing a TFPDP based on a thorough, reflective self-assessment and having taken time to investigate learning resources. Taking an active part in planning spoke placements and other learning activities will give you more confidence to articulate this verbally to those who will support your learning, because you will have generated your own sound evidence base for the learning experiences that you will be asking them for.

Those supporting your learning will benefit from having a well-organised student, who is self-directed, as they will know what you are doing and the purpose of your learning activities, rather than having someone who absorbs their professional caring time by requiring a great deal of direction. You will experience a greater sense of belonging and responsibility within the team to learn the management and decision-making skills that supervisory staff will afford you, if you appear to be well-organised, eager to learn and eager to contribute your own skills as a member of the team. You might like to see the further reading list at the end of the chapter to read more about situated learning and the learning benefits of 'belonging' within the nursing team.

It is now time to construct the content of the third column of the TFPDP. Activity 3.6 will guide you.

Activity 3.6 Team-working to support your learning

Talk to your colleagues and avail yourself of any written or web-based information about your clinical placements and modules that you are studying, so that you know what resources and learning opportunities are available to you.

Consider the students' experiences described in Figure 3.5.

From all of this information, plan to use whatever resources, actions and strategies are appropriate to your own learning objectives, by writing them into the 'Resources, actions and strategies' column of your TFPDP.

As this activity is personal to you, there is no outline answer at the end of the chapter. However, if you need some help with expressing your resources, actions and strategies, have a look at the example in Figure 3.4.

Having identified the resources, and planned your actions and learning strategies, the next part of the development plan allows you to consider how you will know whether these have been effective in helping you to reach your learning objectives.

Planning: identifying evidence of achievement

Planning also includes the recognition of how you will know that you have achieved your learning objectives (the evidence of achievement), so be sure to consider what written, verbal or performed actions will demonstrate to your mentor, personal tutor and yourself that you have achieved the goals at the level set.

You could include the following as evidence of achievement:

- mentor or RN endorsement of official documents – Practice Assessment Competency Documentation, Practice Development Record learning outcomes;
- diary summary written reflections on significant events or learning opportunities, using your own poetic or artistic expressions, and or using a structured reflective model; but always supported by relevant underpinning facts and literature;
- achieving a pass mark or certain percentage in an assessment;
- being offered the job you were interviewed for.

Along with the examples above, you might like to look again at the evidence of achievement offered in Table 2.2 in Chapter 2.

The evidence you choose should be recorded in your TFPDP, as explained in Activity 3.7.

Activity 3.7   Critical thinking

Now that you have identified what might constitute evidence of achievement, write this into the fourth column of your TFPDP, headed 'Success criteria (evidence of achievement)'.

As this activity is personal to you, there is no outline answer at the end of the chapter.

Having completed Activity 3.7, your TFPDP just needs one more planning consideration, as follows.

Planning: setting a review date

- The review date must match the time relation on the learning objective.
- Review should be undertaken each time an interim or final review date is reached. Sometimes a goal will be achieved before the review date; and the review should be written at that time and dated.

- If you miss a review date, make an entry as near to the date as you can and date it contemporaneously.

Be sure to set review dates part way through the time frame, in order to check on your progress with interim objectives that you have set, so that you can celebrate progress and recognise whether there is a need to revise your plan if objectives are not being achieved, or if resources and strategies have not been made available to you; or are simply not available at all and you need to discuss alternative learning strategies with your mentor or personal tutor.

The content of your TFPDP is yours alone and will not look like anyone else's, but the structure should be the same, using the columns from left to right, as the Personal Development Plan uses the systematic stages of action learning.

You should write each column before moving on to the next. When all columns have been considered, go back over and make sure that the content in each column does actually relate to the column heading and is logically connected to each of the other columns. Ensure that the learning objectives are SMART and relate to the overall goal of achieving registration.

Your TFPDP should be endorsed by those supporting your learning, so that the PDP forms a signed agreement of what you will do to help your learning and what will be put in place for you by others. Activity 3.8 will guide you through this process.

Activity 3.8   Team working

Make an appointment to discuss your TFPDP with the team of registered nurses who will support your learning in university and clinical practice, such as your personal tutor, mentor and supervising registrants. As well as endorsing the content that you have written into your TFPDP, it may also prompt them to discuss other learning opportunities, resources, actions and strategies that will be available to you. Remember, this is your plan, personal to your learning objectives, identified from your own self-assessment analysis. Be assertive as to the types of learning opportunities, resources, actions and strategies that you would like to undertake in order to achieve your personal, professional and academic knowledge, skills and attitudes, but also be open to negotiation and suggestion of additional or alternative learning strategies.

Ensure that you obtain signatures and dates agreeing your plan.

As this activity is personal to you, there is no outline answer at the end of the chapter.

Activity 3.8 has resulted in you now having a written TFPDP ready for use to guide you in your transition learning. Keep it with you and use it to guide you on a daily basis so that you have personal drive, can discuss learning achievements with academic staff and can negotiate purposeful learning activities at the beginning of each practice shift.

During implementation of your TFPDP, believe in what you can achieve, work hard and seek constant feedback about your development in order to build confidence. The reward of good quality learning and achievement will become evident when you review your progress. This brings us to the final stage of completing the TFPDP.

Implementation and evaluation

Reviewing achievements and recording results of review

Using the principles of reflection on practice at each of your review dates, will help you to stop, think, look back to where you have come from, think where you are now and look forward to where you can go from here. This reflection should be undertaken with each of the learning objectives that are due for review at that time. It is important to be honest with yourself and give yourself praise for achievements, as well as raising your awareness of improvements needed. In Figures 3.3 and 3.4, I have applied the headings of Borton's (1970, p89) 'reflective sequence', 'What, So What, Now What', to assist you with a review of your achievements (Borton, 1970, p89). As pointed out in Chapter 2, the headings alone may provide only shallow reflection, hence, in Figure 3.4, I have added some specific transition-focussed cues to each heading, in order to provoke deeper, reflective application to what you have learned during the implementation of your TFPDP.

Evaluating your learning thoroughly through completion of the review is essential for appraising what you have achieved and what is still outstanding to carry forward to a new review date. Activity 3.9 assists you to apply the Major (2015) reflective cues within the Borton (1970) reflective sequence.

Activity 3.9 Reflection and critical thinking: evaluating your learning

Undertake a review of your learning *at each of your review dates* using the following cues.

- *What* did I achieve: Looking at my evidence of achievement, did I completely achieve the objective at the standard of performance set, partially achieve it or not achieve it at all?

- *So what* importance does this have for me: What have I learned about myself? Do I need to use a structured reflective model to make sense of the situation?
- *Now what* can I do with this new knowledge, skill or attitude: How can it be used in my future work? How does this enhance my professional work? What benefits will this have for my patients? If I have not achieved the objective, can I carry over anything not completed to the next review date or make a new review date?

You may also have to rethink the learning objectives if they were not achieved. Were they actually specific, measurable, achievable and realistic? Did you perhaps set the interim objectives too high on the taxonomy, or not high enough? Consider whether the resources, actions and strategies were useful – do you need to reconsider what is actually available to you?

Consider whether the evidence of achievement actually provides the level of detail needed to verify your achievements.

Your review evaluation should be undertaken by yourself and shared with your mentors and supervisors as a way of identifying your achievements and needs for further learning. All findings from the review should be written into the final column, or cross-referenced to other documentary evidence of achievement, such as a signed practice assessment document.

Be sure to obtain your assessor's and supervisors' signatures to verify your achievements and any outstanding learning needs identified in the review.

As this activity is personal to you, there is no outline answer at the end of the chapter.

Following Activity 3.9, the process of personal development review for this TFPDP should now be complete. Any outstanding learning could be assigned a new review date, or you may wish to make a new PDP for these.

You may have identified future developmental needs to be written into a preceptorship development plan for your first few months as a registered nurse.

Chapter summary

This chapter has presented a range of reflective models and provided the opportunity for you to engage in structured reflective practice of your own individual transition journey.

Reflective activities have provided the opportunity for you to develop self-awareness of your learning experiences, learning needs and learning achievements, which are a part of the student nurse transition journey towards registration.

(Continued)

(Continued)

The chapter has then encouraged you to use your increased self-awareness to develop TFPDPs, implement them and undertake an evaluative review.

As an aspiring nurse registrant you should now feel well equipped with practical tools to play an active part in managing, and achieving, your own journey towards professional competence for registration.

The reflexivity, which has been encouraged through the activities, has been included in order to provide powerful motivation for you to undertake further self-assessments from multiple perspectives, enabling further professional development planning throughout your professional career.

Activities: brief outline answers

Activity 3.5 Critical thinking (page 67)

Using the learning needs and objectives identified in Figure 3.4:

Self-assessment	Learning objectives
These are the Learning needs identified from self-assessments	**These learning objectives must be SMART**
Having assessed myself against NMC (2010) competency field standard 2, I need to develop my attitude positively towards those patients who have illness related to unhealthy lifestyle choices, by 'respecting people's rights to individual lifestyle choices while trying to promote health and education whenever possible'.	1. During placement seven, I will listen to patients' views and challenge poor health behaviours. 2. By the end of placement seven, I will participate actively in promoting their health and influence change, while justifying the advice given, according to the requirements of competency field standard 2.

1. Start with the time scale: this must be realistic to the time available and any deadlines which have to be met.

Note that the first objective is for achieving *during* placement seven, as a prerequisite of achieving objective two *by the end of* placement seven.

2. The objective must be *specific* to the learning needs identified – note how the objectives directly match the learning needs identified from the self-assessment.

3. The objective must be *measurable* by using a *verb* (doing word or action) that can be seen or heard and should contain *a standard of performance* to be achieved.

The verbs in objective one are – I will *listen* to patients' views and *challenge poor health behaviours*.

This is a required, measurable, performance standard of your course which has to be met – as the self-assessment mentions *NMC competency field standard 2.*

4.   The objective must also be *achievable* and *realistic*.

Is it an achievable and realistic expectation to be able to listen to and challenge patients in this placement? Yes, because this experience is available in every placement.

Objective two also puts all of these SMART components together:

By the end of placement seven, I will *participate actively* in promoting their health and *influence change*, while *justifying* the advice given, according to the *requirements of competency field standard 2*.

Further reading

Chesser-Smyth, P (2013) How to build self-confidence. *Nursing Standard*, 27(52): 64.

This short, easy to read article discusses ways to build your self-belief and confidence during final placements.

Spouse, J (1998) Learning to nurse through legitimate peripheral participation. *Nurse Education Today*, 18(5): 345–51.

This article explains how to increase your sense of belonging within a nursing team so that you can capitalise on the available learning opportunities.

Useful websites

www.businessballs.com/bloomstaxonomyoflearningdomains.htm

Expanded versions of Bloom's, Dave's and Harrow & Simpson's taxonomies of educational objectives, to help you to select the correct action verbs for the levels that you want to achieve.

www.projectsmart.co.uk/brief-history-of-smart-goals.php

For a history of, and some ideas of how to write, SMART objectives.

Chapter 4

Looking after your health and wellbeing during role transition

Leyonie Higgins, Iain Pearson, Melanie Stephens and Mark Widdowson

---

NMC Standards for Pre-registration Nursing Education

This chapter will address the following competencies:

Domain 1: Professional values

Generic competencies

1. All nurses must practice with confidence according to The Code: professional standards of conduct, performance and ethics for nurses and midwives (NMC, 2015), and within other recognised ethical and legal frameworks. They must be able to recognise and address ethical challenges relating to people's choices and decision making about their care, and act within the law to help them and their families and carers find acceptable solutions.

Domain 2: Communication and interpersonal skills

Generic competencies

All nurses must take every opportunity to encourage health-promoting behaviour through education, role modelling and effective communication.

Essential Skills Clusters

This chapter will address the following ESCs:

Cluster: Care, compassion, and communication

1. As partners in the care process, people can trust a newly registered nurse to provide collaborative care based on the highest standards, knowledge and competence.

Entry to the register:

1.1. Is self-aware and self-confident, knows own limitations and is able to take appropriate action.

1.2.   Acts as a role model in promoting a professional image.

1.14.   Uses professional support structures to develop self-awareness, challenge own prejudices and enable professional relationships, so that care is delivered without compromise.

5.   People can trust the newly registered nurse to engage with them in a warm, sensitive and compassionate way.

Entry to the register:

5.11.   Recognises circumstances that trigger personal negative responses and takes action to prevent this compromising care.

5.12.   Recognises and acts autonomously to respond to own emotional discomfort or distress in self and others.

Cluster: Organisational aspects of care

17.   People can trust the newly registered nurse to work safely under pressure and maintain the safety of service users at all times.

Entry to the register:

17.10. Recognises stress in others and provides appropriate support or guidance ensuring safety to people at all times.

17.11. Enables others to identify and manage their stress.

Chapter aims

After reading this chapter you will be able to:

- understand what it is to be physically and emotionally healthy in readiness for the duration of your role transition;
- recognise when you might be physically and/or emotionally unwell during role transition;
- identify factors that can lead to physical and emotional ill health throughout your role transition;
- pinpoint support strategies that will aid in reducing or managing physical and emotional ill health before your role transition.

Introduction

The purpose of this chapter is to increase your awareness of how your personal health and wellbeing can be affected during role transition and in turn how this can influence how you behave and act professionally. The chapter will challenge you, but this will allow you to recognise the signs and symptoms of when you are physically or emotionally unwell in order to help you to take care of yourself when facing the trials and stresses associated with role transition from student nurse to registered nurse.

This chapter will introduce what is meant by health and wellbeing and give you an opportunity to assess your own wellbeing. It then moves on to recognising when you might be physically and/or emotionally unwell. You will have an opportunity to look at the recognisable signs and symptoms of ill health as well as some of the negative habits you may develop when stressed. The chapter then progresses on to identifying and understanding stress before suggesting a range of stressbusting strategies with a focus on building your resilience. Finally, the chapter will focus on accessing support and identifying what support and further resources are available to you.

This chapter starts with a scenario to help demonstrate that you have a responsibility to be aware of your own physical and mental health and address anything that has a negative impact on your practice.

Scenario: Huan the nursing student

Huan is struggling in the final year and has not contacted the university student support services. Huan identifies as a strong person and sees asking for help as a sign of weakness. Huan struggles with excessive worry and being unable to switch off. Recently things have got a lot worse with caring responsibilities at home. Huan is not socialising with classmates, contributing in class, and is attending lectures sporadically. Huan's theory grades have suffered, affecting Huan's self-esteem and confidence.

Huan's mentors have also noted that Huan is afraid to make important decisions, delaying assistance and care to service users. Huan appeared rude and abrupt twice when dealing with patients and family members, and after observing a cardiac arrest Huan had a panic attack and left the shift without informing staff members.

Activity 4.1 asks you to imagine yourself in Huan's shoes and reflect on the implications for your studies and nursing practice.

Activity 4.1 Reflection

1. What would you have done in Huan's situation? Are there any university procedures/support services that could support you?
2. What might the implications be for you in terms of your theory and practice if you continued with/without any change? Are there any penalties that the university might apply?

3. Who might be the best people at your local hospital or community trust to help and advise you? Write down their names and contact details.
4. What might the consequences be for your physical and mental health?

There is an outline answer at the end of the chapter.

As a final year student, Huan may be experiencing stressors similar to those of a newly registered nurse. Early findings regarding third year nursing students from the ongoing REPAIR study conducted by Health Education England found that 'there is a quite a drop-off at the point at which they qualify'.

The *Guardian* reported in 2015 that NHS staff are the most likely public sector workers to feel stressed (60 per cent stressed all or most of the time and 59 per cent saying that they are more stressed this year than last year). Additionally, the number of nurses on stress-related leave and the amount of time taken off equates to 1 in every 29 nurses being off ill with stress (including anxiety and depression) (National Health Executive, 2015). Combining this with the current experiences of students in higher education the picture becomes even more troubling as students accessing counselling services rose 50 per cent in the last five years.

Defining (physical and emotional) health and wellbeing

Concept summary: defining health and wellbeing

As you may well be aware from your nurse education there are both negative and positive definitions of health and wellbeing. As a reminder, negative definitions focus on not having anything wrong with you in relation to disease, disability or injury. Therefore, to feel stressed before and during role transition would not be classed as being ill. However, health and wellbeing is more than absence of an illness. The World Health Organisation's (WHO, 1946, p100) definition of health is *a state of complete physical, mental, and social well-being and not merely the absence of disease or infirmity*. This relates more to why you should look after your health during role transition. Positive definitions, such as the WHO example, demonstrate that health can change from day to day and you will already have seen in practice that some days are more stressful than others; yet, if practice continues to be stressful all the time

(Continued)

(Continued)

your health can become affected. Remember that health and wellbeing also includes social and emotional wellbeing. It is important that newly registered nurses understand the influence their own *culture, traditions, beliefs, patterns, and family interaction* (WHO, 1982, p4) can have on how they manage their health and wellbeing during transition. The Nursing and Midwifery Council (NMC, 2015, p16) identify why physical and emotional wellbeing is important in the section promoting professionalism and trust, stating that all nurses must *maintain the level of health you need to carry out your professional role*. Ignoring your health and wellbeing displays a lack of commitment to professional practice and behaviour.

In order to maintain 'health and wellbeing' it is important to recognise when you are ill.

Recognising ill health in yourself

Deciding when you are too ill (physically or mentally) to continue varies between people; some will immediately go off sick with snuffles and a tickly cough, while others continue on with significant signs and symptoms. Knowing when you are ill and then acting upon this information can often occur only when a friend, family member, colleague, or healthcare practitioner validates the signs and symptoms you might present with. For example, signs of a physical contagious disease are usually synonymous with a pyrexia and tachycardia. Most healthcare practitioners would advise staying off work, taking regular antipyretics and fluids, and returning to work once the pyrexia has resolved after 24 hours. Emotional ill health is more complicated to detect, especially in oneself, and usually time off work is taken only when physical symptoms are present, for example chest pain or palpitations.

Table 4.1 gives a list of signs and symptoms of ill health, both physical and emotional. Look at the lists, could you add any others of your own?

Cognitive symptoms	Emotional symptoms
Memory problems	Moodiness
Poor concentration	Irritability
Poor judgment	Agitation, inability to relax
Seeing only the negative	Feeling overwhelmed
Anxious or racing thoughts	Sense of loneliness and isolation
Constant worrying	Depression or general unhappiness

Physical symptoms	Behavioural symptoms
Aches and pains	Eating too much or too little
Diarrhoea or constipation	Sleeping too much or too little
Nausea, dizziness	Isolating self from others
Chest pain, rapid heartbeat	Procrastinating or neglecting responsibilities
Loss of sex drive	Using alcohol, cigarettes or drugs to relax
Frequently getting ill	Nervous habits (e.g. nail biting, pacing)

Table 4.1   Signs and symptoms of ill health (physical and emotional)

Table 4.1 helps you identify when ill health might be physical or emotional. A simple way to identify why you may be ill is to conduct a health survey.

Activity 4.2   Survey and reflection

Conduct a formal survey about your own health and wellbeing.
There are many online questionnaires about wellbeing, such as the NHS Wellbeing self-assessment (available at: www.nhs.uk/tools/documents/self_assessments_js/assessment.html?&ASid=43&mobile=true&nosplash=true). Complete the questionnaire recording your results. This test should take five minutes to complete and requires you to answer 14 multiple choice questions. It is anonymous and confidential and when completed provides you with a summary about your wellbeing score and evidence based steps to improve your wellbeing; including useful links for more information. Now you have your results, what do you think about your emotional wellbeing? Is there anything you can change?

As this activity is based upon your own reflection, there is no outline answer at the end of the chapter.

Now you have surveyed and reflected on your own health and wellbeing, the next section explores the impact of stress on our lives.

Stress

During role transition you may begin to feel stressed; this is primarily a physical response, which most people see as negative rather than positive (eustress). However, when stressed, the body thinks it is under attack and switches to 'fight or flight' mode, releasing hormones such as adrenaline, cortisol and norepinephrine to prepare the body for physical action. This response causes many reactions, from blood being diverted to muscles to shutting down unnecessary bodily functions such as digestion.

In the today's society the 'fight or flight' mode can help you to survive dangerous situations, such as slamming on the brakes if a person runs in front of your car. During your nurse education, you may have felt stressed during an emergency such as a deteriorating or aggressive patient you have had to deal with. This level of stress has kept you alert to the patient's changing condition and you have sought help promptly.

The challenge is when your body goes into a state of stress in inappropriate situations. When blood flow is only going to the most important muscles needed to fight or flee, brain function is minimised. This response can lead to an inability to 'think straight'; a state that is not useful.

Stress is surprisingly difficult to identify and often takes great self-awareness or indeed someone else to point it out. Even then you may not accept that you are stressed; perhaps because stress is expected as part of your daily nursing life and you have learned to live with it. You assume it is a sign of how busy you are and therefore how accomplished you are in your life. To a certain extent this is ok, it can be a thrilling, engaging and rewarding experience working under pressure (as seen through eustress). However, it can quickly become a problem and a habit. Free time to relax brings feelings of guilt that you should be doing something, you take on more responsibilities than you can handle, and you abandon self-care. You may have noticed this already in situations when your mentor has been so busy they refused to go off the ward for a break each shift and stayed late to complete nursing documentation.

Clearly, it is important to identify the signs and symptoms of stress in order to combat this silent saboteur and take action. Table 4.2 gives a list of some of the thoughts, feelings and behaviours associated with stress (Getselfhelp, 2015).

Thoughts	Emotions
This is too much – I can't cope	Irritable, bad tempered
It's not fair. Someone should be helping me	Anxious
There is too much to do, and too little time	Impatient
I'll never finish	Angry
I have to get this done	Depressed, hopeless
Physical sensations	**Behaviour**
Heart racing, pounding	Crying
Breathing faster	Unsettled, constantly busy, rushing about
Tense muscles – e.g. neck, shoulders, abdomen	Lots on but nothing finished
Hot, sweaty	Sleep disturbances
Headache	Shouting, arguing
Difficulty concentrating	Eating more (or less)
Forgetful	Drinking more
Agitated, restless	Using drugs
Bladder or bowel problems	Smoking more

Table 4.2 Signs and symptoms of stress

Armed with this knowledge you may become better at understanding when either you or someone close to you is experiencing stress.

Activity 4.3 Decision making, reflection, and critical thinking

Consider carrying out a stress test.

Carry out an online stress test such as one provided by the British Association for Counselling and Psychotherapy (2017); this test has ten questions asking you to score yourself against the current pressures of everyday life. It is anonymous and confidential and takes around five minutes to complete. When completed you receive a score, a list of strategies to help you reduce your stress and links to resources you may wish to use. Record your score and reflect on the comments and feedback. What actions should you now take to improve your health and wellbeing?

As this activity is based upon your own reflection, there is no outline answer at the end of the chapter.

When nurses do not manage their stress, it can affect their professional life. The NMC website under hearings and outcomes has several cases where nurses have been stressed and used inappropriate coping mechanisms. Search for a case, read the hearing report and study which parts of the code the panel members refer to when assessing the severity of the charges made due to the nurse's health and wellbeing.

Let's consider health and wellbeing in relation to the use of coping mechanisms.

The concept of self-care within practice and study is important to understand. Nurses are taught to care for others; however, this care cannot and should not take place if you are unable to care for yourself. Exploring the dichotomy between self-care and selfishness reveals that selfishness occurs if you lack concern for or exploit others knowingly and take something with no intention to give it back. Self-care is the appreciation that you are ultimately responsible for taking care of yourself and that if you fail to do this then you are in no position to care for others. Self-care is crucial for the effective management of your wellbeing.

It is worthwhile exploring some other barriers to recognising ill health in yourself; these could be in the form of negative coping theories compounding and worsening the problem. The next section explores some of the main ones to look out for.

Negative coping theories

Martyr complex

Martyr complex (Davis, 1945) is when someone self-sacrifices for a perceived greater good (ultimately at the detriment of their own self-care). During your role transition period this might manifest itself in many ways and, on the surface, this might seem good. However, being a martyr means that you often cannot say 'no' and think you are responsible for everything and everyone. You over-work, communicate poorly and make a big deal about how much you 'have' to do. You never seek help, delegate poorly and expect others to operate at the same high levels as you. Ultimately, this will lead to your own downfall as you become tearful, irritable and operate as a 'victim' with high stress levels until you eventually snap.

Ostrich syndrome

During role transition some students become ostriches to their health and wellbeing with the main thrust of this being denial. It is a passive coping mechanism and generally does not help. You may feel despair, as the longer you don't do it the more you think you can't do it. As humans we can often catastrophise situations that turn out to be not even half as bad as we initially imagined, therefore a lot of the emotional distress is located in the 'not knowing'. For example, you may have gone home and realised you had not handed over some important information and wake up in the night and ring the ward. You then can't sleep as you worry what the night staff will think of you. We all use denial at some point in our lives; however, denial does not resolve the anxiety-producing situation and if overused can lead to psychological distress. It makes sense therefore to deal with situations head-on rather than with your head in the sand.

Perfectionist

As a final year student, you may compare yourself unhelpfully with others, set excessively high standards or take criticism personally even if it is constructive. If you identify with this criterion, then you may be a perfectionist. Perfectionism can often come at the cost of neglecting your relationships and wellbeing, leading to anxiety and depression. Hewitt and Flett (1991) describe three types of perfectionists: *self-oriented* demand the very best of themselves to attain perfection and avoid failure and engage in stringent self-evaluation; *other-oriented perfectionists* set unrealistic standards for others (e.g. partners, children, co-workers) and critically evaluate others' performances; *socially-prescribed perfectionists* believe that others will only like them if they appear to be perfect and believe others evaluate them critically. As a final year student, about to undertake your role transition, you may recognise yourself as one of these.

Social media can have a big influence on the pressure to be perfect, with posts and messages relating to body image, social and student lives. This pressure can lead to feelings of self-doubt and insecurities. You may have the need to constantly prove yourself to others, which can lead to self-defeating aspirations. You may have grown up with social media and may experience the pressure to get 'likes' on your posts or to portray yourself on line as the perfect student, parent, carer and person.

Procrastination

During your role transition you may have a period of preceptorship (see Chapter 7 for more details). During your preceptorship you may be given lots of new knowledge, skills and attitudes to learn and develop. You may find all this overwhelming and this can lead to procrastination. Procrastination can often be mistaken for laziness, but has nothing to do with being lazy. A good definition is *delaying or not completing a task or goal you've committed to, for no valid reason, and instead doing something less important, despite there being negative consequences to not following through on the original task or goal.* Examples could be putting off reading the theory for an extended skill you are about to practise, or revising medications for a test with your preceptor. With a deadline approaching, do you decide that your preceptorship files suddenly need reorganising, you need to tidy your house or there is something on TV that you cannot miss? Procrastination is a strategy to avoid discomfort about doing a task or a goal. It is particularly harmful as it creates more discomfort, preserves our unhelpful rules and assumptions about our abilities and ourselves, makes us more self-critical and piles up tasks. These distressing consequences coupled with the same patterns of behaviour make procrastination even more of an attractive option and thus a vicious cycle is created (Widdowson, 2014). The impact on our emotional wellbeing is significant and the need to implement some practical techniques and adjust our thinking is fundamental, otherwise our emotional wellbeing will suffer (Steel, 2007).

Positive and negative coping mechanisms

As you approach programme completion you may react differently to stressful and anxiety provoking situations. For example, after a busy day at work you may use strategies to help reduce the stress you have been experiencing. Negative coping mechanisms can often make things worse as they are temporary diversions and can affect your physical and emotional health and wellbeing in the long term. Positive coping mechanisms, on the other hand, ground you in the present-day, and by carrying them out they help towards solving the problems that are causing your stress. It is worth mentioning that you can indulge in negative coping mechanisms with limited negative impact, but if their usage is repetitive then it can become destructive. Read the list of negative and positive coping mechanisms given in Table 4.3.

The next section asks you to explore some of the main coping mechanisms you use.

Positive coping mechanisms have advantageous physical and psychological health outcomes. Laughter intensifies the creation of positive emotions, which in turn improves the immune system. Those who laugh off stressful situations are more likely to produce a salivary immunoglobulin that is the first defence in fending off respiratory illnesses (Mahoney, Burroughs, and Lippman, 2002). As well as having a positive impact on physical health, being positive can affect your mental health and reduce stress and depression. The impact of negative coping strategies, however, can include flare-ups of autoimmune illnesses such as psoriasis, Crohn's disease, and lupus to name but a

Positive coping mechanisms	Negative coping mechanisms
Listening to music	Criticising yourself and others
Playing with your children or a pet	Chewing your fingernails
Laughing or crying	Becoming violent or aggressive
Going out with friends	Emotional eating
Taking a long bath	Smoking
Writing, painting, or other creative activities	Drinking alcohol
Exercising	Shouting at your partner, children, or friends
Walking	Taking recreational drugs
Discussing situations with others (colleagues, friends, family)	Mis-using prescription medicine
Gardening	Avoiding friends and family
Practicing mindfulness	Sleeping too much
Writing an action plan or PDP	
Seeking counselling	Excessively watching television

Table 4.3   Positive and negative coping mechanisms

few. Many of the body's systems are affected by negative coping strategies; for example, the gastrointestinal system can be affected by the development of stomach and duodenal ulcers from excessive eating and drinking. Activation of stress hormones can affect the cardiovascular system raising your heart rate, causing chest pain and palpitations, raising your blood pressure and blood lipid levels and decreasing your libido. If not managed, high levels of cholesterol and other fatty substances in the blood can lead to atherosclerosis and even myocardial infarction. Now it is time to consider how you recognise your own health deteriorating.

Activity 4.4   Reflection

Reflect on signs and symptoms of your health deteriorating.

How do you know when your physical health is starting to be compromised, what are the signs and symptoms?

How do you know when your emotional health is starting to be compromised, what are the signs and symptoms?

What feedback or messages do you receive from: family, friends and colleagues?

Review Table 4.3; what positive and negative coping strategies do you utilise?

As this activity is based upon your own reflection, there is no outline answer at the end of the chapter.

Now that you have considered signs and symptoms of physical and emotional ill health it is important to consider strategies for good emotional wellbeing.

Strategies for good emotional wellbeing

No single idea or technique can relieve all your stress, worries or concerns. What often works is openness to different strategies and things that work well for you so that you can use these as you transition into being a registered nurse. It is worth exploring some of the major strategies to manage your emotional wellbeing (there are endless options available with recommended reading at the end of the chapter).

Be organised. Transitioning into professional practice involves managing workloads and prioritising care delivery and you can certainly ease the pressure and sharpen your organisation skills by carrying this into your home life too. Feeling out of control can be one of the main contributors to stress and a lack of orderliness can lead to this. Some quick wins: order or list your concerns and tasks. Use a colour system and alternate mundane tasks with easier or more fun tasks. Think about healthy meals for the week before your weekly shop, are your clothes neatly in the cupboard or scattered around the house? Small changes can make a big overall difference to how you feel.

Letting go of tension. Tension is common during periods of change such as role transition. When unwell, your muscles contract and tense up, this is part of the previously mentioned 'adrenaline response' but over a long period of time this can quite literally be a real pain in the neck. Start by recognising how your body is feeling each day, take a second to work your way down your body thinking about how each part is feeling and make changes. Shoulder massages and diaphragmatic breathing exercises can be useful ways to deal with tension.

Eating, exercise and sleep. Think about your diet, do you usually consume sugary or caffeinated items at busy times? These have a negative effect on your blood sugar levels and after their initial high can leave you irritable and emotional. Consider going decaf, eliminating simple sugars, and replacing them with complex carbohydrates and a range of nutrients/vitamins to ward off illness. How much are you exercising? Exercise reduces your risk of high blood pressure, coronary heart disease, stroke, diabetes and some cancers. It helps manage your weight, reducing your risk of obesity and prevents mental health problems through boosting your mood. Start small, you do not have to join the gym. Finally, how is your sleep? Not getting enough sleep can significantly affect stress. Resilience levels are reduced and to combat tiredness we are more likely to reach for sugars and caffeine. Try to ensure you get enough sleep and make sure it is the rule rather than an exception. Using a phone or computer device before bed prevents your brain from releasing melatonin, the hormone that tells you it's time to sleep. Try switching off your device an hour before you go to sleep; you will fall asleep faster. If your environment is not conducive to sleep, make changes. Even if this means using earplugs to reduce noise, it is worth doing!

Worrying less. It is common for nursing students to feel insecure about their competence and ability to step into working life. Uncontrollable worrying is very unproductive and tends to generate more emotional distress. If you have an unhelpful attitude to perfection, try the following: have a social media 'detox', remember many pictures, videos, statuses, tweets, snapchats have been altered with filters. Social media is a constructed reality; it doesn't reflect real life – the perfect life doesn't exist. Change your focus; try thinking about the process, 'how and why you are doing things right now' rather than the outcome 'what you might achieve'. Avoid judging, overthinking, regretting or feeling guilty about past events that you cannot change, think instead about how the past can help improve the present and future. Practice thinking and behaving more flexibly: identify three different approaches to a goal, outcome or person, try using words such as 'alternatively', 'possibly', 'sometimes', 'compromise' and 'occasionally'. Consider the words you use to describe yourself and others, try and exchange negative words for positive ones (for example, instead of telling yourself you 'should' do something, say you 'choose' to); use softer words, be less harsh on yourself. Being perfect does not always make you happy; the perfect person, nurse or life does not exist.

Meditation and mindfulness. They offer a useful option for emotional distress and are easily applicable. Mindfulness focusses on letting go of distractions, particularly past regrets, low mood, and pre-empts how a situation may pan out, reducing anxiety. Staying 'in the present' is key and could be as simple as focussing on sensory elements such as touch, sight, hearing, smell and taste. This can be difficult initially, but practice improves this, and it becomes a very valuable tool to prevent worrying; just like a muscle, your mind needs exercising. Try 'worry postponement'. Rather than carrying your problems with you throughout the day, allocate a specific time to process all your worries. Park your worries as they emerge during the day and wait for this time. Then sit down and review them, perhaps some will even have subsided.

Interpersonal effectiveness. Relationships can be a great cause of stress. Communication is at the centre of this and involves good listening skills. If you are a poor listener, then this can affect your role transition to the extent where you have less effective relationships with physicians, nurses and patients, work less confidently and have more stress in your life. Listening is a complex skill, it is about non-verbal communication such as nodding, facial expressions and showing genuine interest in what the other person says. Identify your communication style; passive communicators are compliant, submissive, self-critical and operate from a 'you're ok, I'm not' viewpoint. They give in to others, don't get what they want, are self-deprecating and feel miserable. Aggressive communicators are sarcastic, patronising, and disrespectful of others. They offend others and feel angry and resentful. Assertive communicators however are firm, polite, send clear messages and are respectful of themselves and others. Consequently, they have good relationships with others, are happy with outcomes and happy to compromise. Working to become an assertive communicator would help with your transition into professional practice.

After making necessary changes you could still be struggling to work out how to make your life healthier, this is where it is worth considering talking therapies to help you before or during your role transition. A range of studies have shown that talking therapies can be significantly effective for a range of mental health problems including anxiety and depression; to view these studies you can visit the British Association for Counselling and Psychotherapy (BACP) website.

There are many types of psychotherapy and counselling available, however the most important predictor of a positive outcome from talking therapies is the strength of the relationship between you and the therapist. Through counselling, you can explore and gain clarity of your situation and develop a deeper understanding of yourself. You can identify useful behaviour changes and develop new coping skills. Accessing therapies can be organised through your GP or self-referral on the NHS, through charities, local organisations, university services or privately. It is important to check credentials of private services using the BACP online find a therapist tool. If you do see a therapist, make sure it is someone friendly, professional and who you feel comfortable opening up to.

If you have identified that you are stressed during your role transition you may wish to address this with the following activity.

Activity 4.5   Decision making and reflection

Dealing with stress.

Choose one activity on how to deal with stress, carry out the activity for 6 weeks, repeat the stress test and also reflect on the effect; ask family and friends for their feedback too.

As this activity is based upon your own decision-making processes and reflection, there is no outline answer at the end of the chapter.

As you start to reduce stress levels by carrying out a stress reducing activity or identifying your negative coping mechanisms you may start to learn more about yourself and how emotionally aware you are now becoming.

Emotional intelligence

The concept of emotional intelligence has become popular in recent years. Emotional intelligence involves the ability to accurately identify what you are feeling at any given moment, and then to think about and reflect upon your emotions and use these creatively to guide your thinking and actions. Emotional intelligence also includes the capacity to regulate your emotions appropriately. Nurses with high levels of emotional intelligence have strong social skills and a capacity to understand others and respond in a helpful way to their emotions. Moreover, high levels of emotional intelligence have been associated with an increased ability to handle stress and reduced levels of burnout. A high level of emotional intelligence is undoubtedly beneficial during role transition. Fortunately, emotional intelligence can be developed and the suggestions in this chapter will help increase your emotional intelligence. Emotional intelligence and psychological resilience are linked. Increased emotional intelligence improves resilience and activities aimed at developing resilience in turn have a positive effect on emotional intelligence.

What is resilience?

Resilience is the ability to manage hard times in our lives, and 'bounce back' or cope with setbacks, disappointment and hurt; your resilience may be tested at times during your final year. Resilience is a key skill to ensuring good mental health and involves developing the ability to hang on in there or stick with it even when you really want to give up. Having good self-esteem, self-compassion and self-confidence, being more able to cope with stress, manage strong feelings, adapt to stressful situations and develop effective problem-solving strategies, are all traits and abilities of a person with resilience. During your role transition, you may be required to set realistic goals that include resilience and plan how you are going to achieve them as resilience is something that anyone can develop at any time in their lives. Table 4.4 provides ten ways to build your resilience during your final year.

1. *Make connections.* Strengthen good supportive relationships with your family, friends and colleagues.

2. *Avoid seeing crises as insurmountable problems.* Stressful events are a natural part of life – we all experience them occasionally. When times get tough, it's easy to see each new problem as something that's testing your ability to cope. While you can't change events, you can change how you respond to them.

3. *Accept that change is a part of life.* Learning to accept circumstances that cannot be changed or are out of your control. Learn to revise goals in light of circumstances and situations.

4. *Move towards your goals.* There is no point having goals if you don't work on them. Each step you take (no matter how small) moves you that bit further towards achieving your goals.

5. *Take decisive action.* Whenever situations get difficult, resilient people take action to deal with or change them. Being passive or pretending the problem doesn't exist is an ineffective strategy.

6. *Look for opportunities for growth and self-discovery.* In each difficult or painful situation, there is always something positive you can take from it. It might be learning something new about yourself, or an increased sense of what is really important in life.

7. *Build your self-confidence.* Working on increasing your self-confidence has a wide range of benefits, including enhancing your ability to bounce back from adversity.

8. *Develop a long-term perspective* (seeing the problem as being just one phase of your life). This means not blowing things out of proportion or 'catastrophising'. Take a broader view and feel grateful for the good things you have in your life.

9. *Remain optimistic.* Stay hopeful and have a positive outlook on life.

10. *Take care of your body.* Be sure to look after both your physical and mental health.

Table 4.4   Ten ways of building resilience

Source: American Psychological Association (2016).

Consider your circle of control

It is acknowledged that resilient, proactive people focus their time and energies on things that they can control or influence; a positive focus on the circle of influence enlarges your circle of control (Covey, 1989; see Figure 4.1). If you have a reactive focus on things you cannot influence or control you are neglecting the things you can control; by focussing on the things you can control your life will improve. These are essential skills to develop before and during role transition.

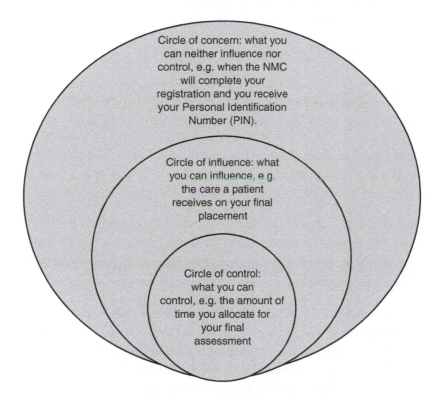

Figure 4.1   Circles of influence, control and concern

The Royal College of Nursing (RCN) leadership programme offers a tool based on Covey's model to help you organise your worries into the three circles. By doing this you can begin to have an impact on the concerns you can influence and let go of those you cannot, becoming a proactive and effective newly registered nurse. Try making a note of your main issue from your role transition and then explore what things you can control and influence, for example your words, ideas, effort, behaviour, emotions and actions. Then consider what things you can neither influence nor control, for example other people's emotions, words, actions, mistakes.

Accessing support

As a student nearing registration, you may contemplate the effects of losing the support mechanisms that were in place during your undergraduate studies. Feeling overwhelmed, fear of failure and stressed at the prospect of professional accountability can affect your mental health. Mood change is normal but it is important to act if your mood starts to negatively impact your life, is different from usual, or there is a constant feeling of anxiety.

Before you move into professional practice, it is recommended to make a change, and this could mean speaking to your GP. Going to your GP may cause some anxiety but it is important to reframe this; if your leg was broken, you would see a doctor. Taking early timely action often leads to a better outcome.

It is now worth considering your support networks.

Who would you talk to? It is always better to have a voice or face-to-face conversation (e.g. Skype) rather than messaging. Write down the name and contact numbers of two trusted people you can talk to when you are worried, anxious or stressed.

Are you registered with your local GP service? Access NHS choices to find and register with a local practice. Write down the telephone number, location, how to get there, the appointment booking system, plus what to do if you want a same day or telephone appointment.

Where is the nearest walk-in centre? If you are experiencing physical health symptoms, you may be able to get treatment at your local walk-in centre. Nurses provide a range of treatments for minor illnesses and injuries; they may also provide smoking cessation support. Write down opening and closing times, location and directions to the centre.

Do you have caring responsibilities? Identify one or two people who can help you for a short time; this may be so that you can attend appointments, e.g. GP or counselling services, or spend some time on positive self-care. Write down their names and contact details. Ensure that you have discussed with them whether they can be contacted at any time (night or day) or just at certain times, do they need to be left care instructions, how will they get to you, how long will it take them? Will they require any form of payment? You will need to consider your caring responsibilities as a registered nurse; e.g. who will take over your caring responsibilities if school is closed due to snow?

What activities are available in your local area? Exercise doesn't have to cost you anything. Use the internet to find your nearest park or local free outdoors gym. Most universities have reduced student fees to join their sports facilities; some offer the opportunity to try out new activities at a discounted cost. Access the internet to find your local council leisure/sports/fitness centre; they are often cheaper than commercial companies and offer the same great facilities.

Chapter summary

By reading this chapter, we hope that you will be able to comprehend more about your physical and mental health. By completing the reading and activities you should now be able to recognise when you might be physically and/or emotionally unwell; identify factors that can lead to physical and emotional ill health; and describe support strategies that will help reduce or manage your physical and emotional ill health during your role transition and for the rest of your nursing career.

Activities: brief outline answers

Activity 4.1 Reflection (page 80)

1. Huan could start to fail theory and practice assessments, impacting classification and ability to pass the programme. Huan could be subject to the universities 'Fitness to practice' procedure. All students whose programme of study leads to registration on a health or social care register must abide by their university fitness to practice principles, standards and procedure.

2. If Huan had assessments, the university's 'mitigating circumstances' procedure could have been accessed. All universities have a procedure in place as a part of their Academic Regulations that students can access to ensure exceptional circumstances can be mitigated for. It would also never be too late for Huan to register and make an appointment with the local GP surgery to discuss their emotional and physical health. This is particularly relevant if evidence of their circumstances is needed for mitigation. Finally, Huan would benefit from informing their personal tutor and university counselling service as soon as possible of their difficulties, particularly if their mental and physical health problems were showing no signs of changing without intervention.

3. Placement support: Current mentor, Ward/Unit or Community Team manager, a member of staff from the Practice Education Team. If Huan was a newly registered nurse: their Preceptor, Ward/Unit/Community Team Manager, the Occupational Health Department.

4. See the section on stress (page 83).

Further reading

Davis, M, Eshelman, M and McKay, ER (2008) *The Relaxation and Stress Reduction Workbook.* Oakland, CA: New Harbinger Publications.

An accessible and comprehensive step by step instructions for a range of relaxation techniques for effective stress management.

Elkin, A (1999) *Stress Management for Dummies.* Foster City, CA: IDG Books.

A book full of useful techniques looking at managing stress. Either follow sequentially or dip in to find practical techniques that work for you.

Gupta, S (2008) *Stress Management A Holistic Approach.* London: Subodh Gupta.

Following a 5-step strategy, this book sets out to raise a holistic awareness of stress and find solutions.

Harris, R (2008) *The Happiness Trap: Stop struggling, start living.* Available at: www. thehappinesstrap.com/

Taking a mindfulness-based approach based on the five principles of acceptance and commitment therapy, this book provides techniques to reduce stress and worry.

Williams, C (2012) *Overcoming Anxiety, Stress, and Panic: A five areas approach* (3rd edn). Boca Raton, FL: Taylor & Francis.

Excellent, clear user-friendly format using a five area approach model of intervention for anxiety, stress and panic.

Williams, M and Penman, D (2011) *Mindfulness: A practical guide to finding peace in a frantic world.* London: Piatkus.

Based on mindfulness-based cognitive behavioural therapy, this book is useful for those who are struggling to keep up with the demands of the modern world.

Useful websites

www.nhs.uk/change4life

Information on eating well, exercise and healthy living.

www.nutrition.org.uk/

British Nutrition Foundation; you can find information here about why good nutrition and lifestyle choices are important for your health and wellbeing.

www.getselfhelp.co.uk/stress.htm

Overcoming and understanding stress, a good basic introduction.

www.youtube.com/watch?feature=player_embedded&v=I6402QJp52M

The single most important thing you can do for your stress – video on how to manage stress.

www.mentalhealth.org.uk/a-to-z/m/mindfulness

A good introduction to mindfulness.

www.itsgoodtotalk.org.uk/therapists

The BACP Find a Therapist tool to aid you in finding the right therapist.

Useful apps

Moodtrack diary: a free app to track your moods anytime, anywhere. You can track as much as you want, share your thoughts or keep them private and reflect on your moods to learn more about yourself.

Headspace: offers a free introductory series with ten sessions for 10 minutes each that will enable you to start to obtain a happier, healthy life.

YouTube: you can search for useful resources on managing stress, indoor exercises, mindfulness, meditation, yoga and Tai Chi.

Chapter 5

Learning theory for personal and professional development

Jacqueline Leigh and Tyler Warburton

NMC Standards for Pre-registration Nursing Education

This chapter will address the following competency:

Domain 1: Professional values

Generic standard for competence: All nurses must act first and foremost to care for and safeguard the public. They must practise autonomously and be responsible and accountable for safe, compassionate, person-centred, evidence-based nursing that respects and maintains dignity and human rights. They must show professionalism and integrity and work within recognised professional, ethical and legal frameworks. They must work in partnership with other health and social care professionals and agencies, service users, their carers and families in all settings, including the community, ensuring that decisions about care are shared.

Essential Skills Clusters

This chapter will address the following ESCs:

Cluster: Care, compassion and communication

1. As partners in the care process, people can trust a newly registered graduate nurse to provide collaborative care based on the highest standards, knowledge and competence.

1.9. Is self-aware and self-confident, knows own limitations and is able to take appropriate action.

Cluster: Organisational aspects of care

12. People can trust the newly registered graduate nurse to respond to their feedback and a wide range of other sources to learn, develop and improve services.

(Continued)

(Continued)

12.6.   Actively responds to feedback.

14.   People can trust the newly registered graduate nurse to be an autonomous and confident member of the multi-disciplinary or multi-agency team and to inspire confidence in others.

14.7.   Challenges the practice of self and others across the multi-professional team.

15.   People can trust the newly registered graduate nurse to safely delegate to others and to respond appropriately when a task is delegated to them.

15.5.   Recognises and addresses deficits in knowledge and skill in self and others and takes appropriate action.

Chapter aims

After reading this chapter you will be able to:

* discuss the relevance of understanding how you learn to transition;
* explain key learning theories relating to transition and your learning journey;
* understand your learning preferences and strategies to improve your learning;
* plan learning strategies for your transition from student to newly registered nurse, including learning from work and utilising existing role models.

Introduction

One of our defining features as human beings is an enormous capacity to learn new things, be they skills, behaviours or bodies of knowledge. It is something that starts at birth, continues to the grave and shapes our lives at every point in between. This chapter will explore the importance of understanding how you learn and how this knowledge can be used to support your transition from student to newly registered nurse. This chapter will begin by introducing two scenarios based around two student nurses who are at different stages of their nursing programme and who demonstrate similarities and different preferences for learning.

Throughout this chapter, you will be provided with opportunities and learning activities to draw on these two scenarios and as the chapter progresses you will be introduced to a third and final scenario in order to make sense of the range of learning theories and how they can be applied to your role transition.

Theories include behaviourism, social learning theory, cognitive theories of learning as well as a review of the social aspects of learning. The final section is about understanding your own learning preferences, enabling you to optimise your learning in the future.

Consider the following two scenarios

Scenario 1

Alex is a 22-year-old third year student nurse who is dedicated to study and has good support from family in relation to completing the study necessary to gain a degree in nursing. Alex has successfully passed on the first attempt all practice based assessments and NMC competencies. However, Alex has not passed two of the theoretical assignments at the first attempt. Alex reflects on approaches to completing the assignments and on the written feedback provided by the marker and academic supervisor. The written feedback and verbal comments Alex has received include: seeking minimal support from the academic supervisor; not effectively planning time to study; not making the most out of feedback from previous academic assignments.

Alex enjoyed and expressed a preference for the formative group presentation that formed part of the academic programme – this was a new form of learning and assessment for Alex. Alex finds the lecture the least useful method of learning.

Scenario 2

Taylor is a second year student nurse who entered nursing following a 10 year career in retail. Taylor describes a preference for learning in small groups and needing time to reflect on information before responding to a question or joining in group work with peers. Although disorganised when planning study time, Taylor enjoys reading journal papers and critiquing the evidence base. Taylor finds that a mind map or visual display helps make sense of the complex information found in the papers. Taylor enjoys the online learning and finds the lecture the least useful method of learning. Similar to Alex, introduced in scenario 1, Taylor enjoys learning in clinical practice and has successfully met all of the NMC competencies required so far. Mentor feedback includes effectively communicating with a patient who was hard to engage in conversation with and demonstrating an ability to practice clinical skills under the supervision of a registered nurse.

The importance of understanding how you learn

This chapter has started with the above scenarios to help set the context of two student nurses' reflections on their preferences for learning. As can be seen from the scenarios, Taylor and Alex have different preferences for learning both in the ways they learn and in the settings in which learning takes place. This first activity will explore the concept of learning.

Activity 5.1   Reflection

When you hear the term 'learning', what do you think of? What key words spring to mind and what do these words mean to you?

As this is based on your experience there is only a brief outline answer at the end of this chapter.

An individual's capacity to learn can at times be readily observable, such as a baby's first steps or the achievement of an academic award. At other times its influence can be significantly less obvious; for example, influencing interpersonal relationships, self-belief and developing an understanding of who we are. Despite its overwhelming influence on people's lives, it is something that is often taken for granted and very prone to false assumptions.

One of these often-held false assumptions is that an individual's capacity to learn is either a fixed trait, or a trait that can only be changed within a narrow margin. This often goes hand in hand with the ideology that some people are just better at learning than others. As a result there is the belief that some people are innately more likely to achieve greater things than others. It is indeed true that capacity to learn is not the same for everyone; as with any ability there is likely to be a degree of variance between one person and the next. Furthermore, some individuals will demonstrate a greater aptitude or preference for certain skills or areas of study. Referring back to Alex in scenario 1, Alex expressed a preference for the formative group presentation that formed part of the academic programme. This was opposed to attending a lecture, which was identified as Alex's least useful approach for learning.

In reality, however, it is perhaps more likely that the gap between individual capacities is significantly smaller than you think. The assumption noted above can be very problematic to learners, particularly if you have had poor learning experiences previously. Your own experience will tell you that your capacity to learn can vary greatly and is dependent upon a host of different factors such as enablers and barriers.

This next activity provides you with the opportunity for you to explore your enablers and barriers to successful learning.

Having explored what might help or hinder your learning we now look at learning habits.

Of all assumptions (true or false) that you can make about your learning the most debilitating is perhaps that you do not need to think about it. Learning just happens. In many respects it does, but it might not always happen in the way and indeed quantity desired. By taking charge of it and understanding it, you can optimise it. Transitioning from a student to a newly registered nurse marks a significant milestone in your

Activity 5.2   Critical thinking

While attending your undergraduate nursing programme, consider something that you found easy to learn and something that you found hard. This may relate to theory or clinical practice or both. What factors contributed to your learning or to how easy or hard you found the learning? What were your barriers?

A brief outline answer can be found at the end of this chapter.

career. To get to that stage has taken you a tremendous amount of learning in university, clinical practice and life in general. This is not an end point; it is the start of the next journey. The challenge now is to reconfigure your learning practices to get you through the next stage.

In your learning journey so far you may have developed a variety of learning habits and techniques within the educational setting that will help with your transition; others, however, will not and need to be adjusted or abandoned. This is where having an understanding of learning theory will prove invaluable. It will enable the identification and selection of the most efficient learning habits and techniques so you can make the most of your learning.

This next activity will help you to explore and identify learning habits in relation to a defined situation through using the two scenarios about Alex and Taylor.

Activity 5.3   Decision making

Consider scenarios 1 and 2 introduced to you at the start of this chapter and then list the range of learning habits reported on by Alex and Taylor. From your list of identified habits place a tick next to those habits that have supported each student's learning. *A brief outline answer can be found at the end of this chapter.*

Think about a situation either in the university or clinical setting whereby you have learned something new or different. For this situation, produce a list of your identified learning habits, placing a tick next to those habits that you feel supported your learning. You can repeat this for different situations, in particular try and explore something that you achieved in the end, but you found it very difficult to get there. What kept you going throughout this and stopped your giving up? How did you eventually conquer it?

As this activity is based on your own experiences there is no outline answer at the end of the chapter; however, you will be asked to refer to this list as part of Activity 5.6.

Having thought about what helped your learning, you are next introduced to some of the key learning theories and how they could apply to your role transition. Scenarios 1 and 2 are again referred to specifically to help you to contextualise the learning theories and these are supplemented with activities for you to complete. A final third scenario will help you to understand the differences between the behaviourist and cognitive theories of learning.

Consideration of different learning theories

Before engaging in this next part of the chapter it is worth reflecting on your definition of learning. This next activity provides the opportunity to do this.

Activity 5.4 Evidence based practice and research

Write down your definition of learning. Next, search using journals or the internet to compare definitions. Identify any similarities or differences.

A brief outline answer can be found at the end of this chapter.

It is important to point out that many individuals will have very strongly held views regarding how to learn. The act of learning is not a simple and straight forward process. It is complex, multifaceted and context bound. As a result of this there exists a host of different theories and ideologies seeking to explain how learning occurs and what factors promote and inhibit it. There is a temptation to find a learning theory you can relate to and use it exclusively to analyse, plan and evaluate learning. This is a poor approach to take as the different theories are based on very different models and ideologies. Just as viewing an object from different angles allows you to see different features of the object, appraising your learning practices using different theories also provides a diversity of insights to explore.

In many instances people's personal view may mimic or at least fit with, the basic tenets of key learning theories. At other times there may appear to be an internal or innate conflict to such theories. This can be challenging for an individual who is seeking to analyse learning practices, particularly when faced with ideas that challenge a deeply held view. This is often a key aspect of the self-evaluation process that needs to be engaged with using a high level of critical maturity. The important thing to remember is that the different theories are conceptual models to be used in the analysis, exploration and discussion of learning.

Learning theories are often described in chronological order based upon when they first emerged into the scholarly literature. This can be helpful as it allows you to conceptualise them in terms of the commonly held beliefs and assumptions at the time in which they were developed. This chronology does not in itself make more recent theories better in comparison to their older counterparts. The actual space of time between many of those that are still popular today is very short. It is merely a representation of how the trends in thinking and conceptualising have changed over time. It is possible that as you explore your own learning you may find value in the many different theories and use different components to support your personal transition.

Next you will be introduced to a range of theories of learning and after the last theory you will be introduced to an activity whereby you will reflect on how useful each could be when applied to your transition from student to newly registered nurse. To help contextualise the theories you will be asked to draw on the scenarios of the two students, Alex and Taylor, introduced to you at the start of this chapter. A further scenario will be presented to you (scenario 3), to help demonstrate the difference between the behaviourist and cognitive theories of learning.

Behaviourist theories of learning

One of the earliest theories of learning to be popularised is behaviourism. Emerging in the early twentieth century and advanced by researchers such as John Watson, Burrhus Skinner and Ivan Pavlov (Kellogg, 2002). Two of the most basic and key concepts within behaviourism are those of 'classical conditioning' (Pavlov, 1960) and 'operant conditioning' (Skinner, 1969). Both of these concepts concern themselves with looking at the association between a stimulus and a response. One of the main criticisms of behaviourism is that it is too simplistic and focusses only on observable actions. To some degree this may be true but this does not invalidate its relevance, particularly when reviewing your own practices.

Operant conditioning is very often misrepresented as being a dichotomy between positive reinforcement (reward) and punishment (often incorrectly termed 'negative reinforcement'). This is not the case, the true theory of operant conditioning is a little richer. Positive reinforcement is as it is often portrayed, the reward of a particular behaviour. This can be a conscious act by someone, such as providing a reward of some kind when the desired behaviour is displayed. Referring back to scenario 2 with Taylor the second year student nurse, it may for example be circumstantial, such as getting a positive outcome after trying a different approach to communicating with a patient who is hard to engage in conversation with. The reward thus increases Taylor's likelihood of using that behaviour again.

The opposite of positive reinforcement is punishment, not to be confused with negative reinforcement discussed below. Punishment is not necessarily as severe as it sounds from its label. It is essentially anything that is negative enough to discourage the action or behaviour that caused it from being issued. So in our communication example with

Taylor, they may have attempted to start a difficult conversation with a patient or team member that results in the individual becoming more withdrawn from the engagement or getting upset. Thus, in the future, Taylor would be significantly less likely to employ that approach.

One of the key things to remember with the operant conditioning theory is it works equally well to reinforce undesirable behaviour as it does desirable behaviour. This is particularly noted in the instance of negative reinforcement. Taking the time to observe the daily practices and routines in the work place can highlight many examples of this. Particularly when individuals have found that engaging in a sub-optimal approach to something goes unnoticed but enables them to get though their workload quicker. An example might be if a nurse distributes the medication for all of their patients into pots at the start of the day for breakfast, lunch and teatime medicines rounds. They leave these on the side in the treatment room to be distributed at the set time. This is evidently an unsafe and unprofessional practice, but if it is left unchallenged (punished) it could continue as the reward is saving them time later. Negative reinforcement is where the likelihood of repeating a behaviour/action is increased (reinforced) by the removal of something unpleasant or the avoidance of punishment. Taking this example further, the nurse is putting patients at risk of harm and could be punished in a number of ways. This could include being directly challenged by a colleague, facing disciplinary action from their employer or being referred to the NMC for professional misconduct and struck off the register if found guilty. Negative reinforcement could potentially occur at any stage; for example if the employer was seen to be lenient in the face of similar instances of unsafe practice or if the NMC disciplinary process came to be viewed as ineffective. As the example shows, effective and appropriate punishment is vital in preventing negative reinforcement from occurring and explains why a robust set of effective and well-enforced rules is central to safe nursing practice.

So as can be seen, behaviourism can help explain how and why different behaviours and practices are adopted by individuals. It does not, however, fully explain all the learning you undertake and ignores a few key aspects of effective learning.

Social learning theory

Following on from the concept of operant conditioning is social learning theory (Bandura, 1977b). Bandura (1977b) described this theory following his famous bobo doll experiment. This theory built on that of operant conditioning by demonstrating that particular behaviours and factors can be vicariously 'reinforced' by observing the results gained by others – essentially suggesting that witnessing someone else getting rewarded for a particular action makes you more likely to engage in that action. Likewise, witnessing punishment discourages it. Many people would term this role-modelling.

The notion of role-modelling is yet again a concept whose face value belies its intricacy. It is easy to see how witnessing another person's actions get rewarded will make such action more desirable to replicate. Take for example Alex in scenario 1 who observed other students and then participated in the formative group presentation. Role modelling is not as simplistic as being presented with a good example, there are several stages one must progress through before modelling behaviour. These stages are set out in Table 5.1.

- Attention – this is where an individual decides who to model their behaviour on; this will be influenced by how potential models are viewed and is influenced by things such as perceived power, seniority, recognised mentor and how many followers they already have.

- Retention – during this stage an individual will observe the behaviours and actions of their potential models and store them for later use.

- Reproduction – the individual will now start to practise the observed behaviours; these may be very subtle at first with them just testing out small components in relatively safe environments.

- Motivation – this stage is where the individual will review the feedback they are getting from their new actions/behaviours. The more positive they find this feedback, the more likely they are to adopt them.

Table 5.1   Stages of modelling behaviour

Source: adapted from Bandura (1977b).

The time it takes to progress through these stages will depend on the situation. A very important factor to keep in mind as a developing practitioner is why you have chosen to model the behaviour of a particular individual or individuals. As can be seen from the description in the 'attention' phase, decisions around this point are likely to be heavily influenced by things such as personal ideals, culture and even the media. Being very aware of what has drawn you to seek to model particular behaviours can be illuminating and in some cases help you to realign your efforts towards more achievable or professionally desirable role-models. Practising within the NMC Code (NMC, 2015) may influence your decisions when selecting a role model. As with the conditioning theories above, it will be useful for you to reflect and summarise how you could apply this theory to your transition and your role as newly registered nurse.

Cognitive theories of learning

One of the major limitations of the behaviourist theories was that they did not concern themselves with the internal processes involved with learning (Butts and Rich, 2014). As noted when exploring learning theories in general, this is more of a defining feature of the standpoint of the period in which they were first developed, as opposed to an oversight on the researcher's part. One of the major challenges a newly registered nurse faces when dealing with unpredictable and unique situations and events is that no amount of pre-qualifying education can prepare you for every eventuality. Yet safe effective practice is contingent on your ability to act in such uncertainty as noted in the example in scenario 3. In order to explore how this happens, there needs to be a consideration of the internal processes involved in learning. Specifically, the ability to formulate mental models of the world around you so that you can choose the best course of action. This is termed 'Gestalt thinking' (Kellogg, 2002).

As with behaviourism, 'cognitive' theories of learning are a relatively blanket term for a host of different theories and concepts. Collectively they all share a very common premise: *people are thinking entities capable of modelling scenarios in an abstract sense* (Warburton, Houghton and Barry, 2016, p43). What this means, is that within your mind you are able to construct a mental representation of the world around you with which to test ideas and potential approaches. So, for example, with the scenario 3 below Alex instinctively considered various alternative courses of action and their likely outcomes before undertaking the task. This allowed Alex to select the course of action that, based on their understanding of the factors associated with the situation, would give the best outcome.

Scenario 3

Imagine that a registered nurse has requested that you explain to a patient and their relatives that there is going to be a significant delay before they are seen by the multi-professional team. This is not something you have had to do previously and nor is it something you have witnessed another member of staff perform. Nevertheless you are still able to undertake the task based on your knowledge and understanding of various different factors and issues associated with the allocated task. However, this is not undertaken blindly or without thought. When approaching the task you would not simply walk over and start the conversation with the patient and their relatives. Instead, and very instinctively you would first think about the task, running over several courses of action in your head to see which you think would get the best result. This may take only moments to do, but it would enable you to take more purposeful action.

Looking at learning from a cognitive perspective shifts the focus from that of reacting to the world around you – towards thinking about and planning your actions. The limitation is that your mental models of the world around you are only as good as your understanding of it. Experience can provide an enormous advantage. The more experience you have of a particular situation or phenomenon the more you have to draw upon when constructing a mental representation of it. However, experience alone is not enough. To truly understand and learn from those experiences, you need to reflect upon them. As a healthcare professional you are likely used to the concept of reflection and indeed this is covered in more detail in Chapter 3. For the purpose of this discussion around learning the term will be used fairly loosely.

David Kolb developed a learning model to describe this process known as the experiential learning cycle (Kolb, 1984). The model represents a cyclical process that Kolb (1984) argued must be undertaken in order for effective learning to take place. Kolb's cycle is provided in Figure 5.1.

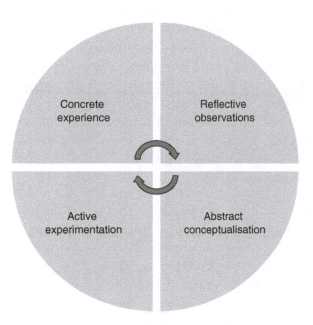

Figure 5.1 Kolb diagram

It is possible to enter the cycle at any point but most people find it easier to understand by starting with a *concrete experience*; such as undertaking a dressing change, patient assessment or interpersonal interaction. Following this experience, the individual will make reflective observations about how it went, noting good points and bad points, or perhaps points where the reality did not meet their expectations. These observations result in the prior understanding being reviewed in light of the new information. This is termed *abstract conceptualisation*. For example, concluding that not all patients respond in the same way to a standards approach or that a certain dressing is not always the best for a wound. This then leads into the *active experimentation* phase whereby new ideas are conceptually or practically tested in order to see whether they work. This leads back around to the concrete experience phase once more.

How quickly one goes through the cycle will vary based on factors such as the task itself, the time you have to reflect, frequency of exposure and so forth. What is perhaps important to understand in relation to this, is that it demonstrates that simple repetition does not constitute learning. Reflecting on past experiences and using mental models to explore different ideas and options are essential to learning. The notion of Gestalt thinking allows the construction of conceptual models of 'what if' scenarios to explore without the need for first-hand experience.

Social aspects of learning

As with all theories, cognitive theories of learning are not without their limitations. Like their behaviourist predecessors, they largely originate from a time in which the 'positivist ideology' of the absolute truth was prevalent (Fosnot, 2005). Consequently, the methods used to develop them relied very heavily on statistical analysis of observations to generate new knowledge. There was no interest in the interpretation of those observations or the possibility of having multiple valid interpretations of a phenomenon. More recent learning theories such as 'constructivism' place a higher regard on the individual's interpretation of their experiences and suggest that learners will interpret new knowledge and understanding through the lens of their current understanding of the world. Thus this may result in differing yet equally valid interpretations.

Another key limitation of many of the earlier theories of learning was its initial disregard for the social factors that influence learning. This is perhaps due to the very late adoption of sociology as an academic discipline, particularly in Great Britain and the United States (Boronski and Hassan, 2015). The 'attentive' phase of behaviour modelling proposed by Bandura alludes to the influence social factors play in what and how people learn, but it does not adequately expand on this. Take for example Alex and Taylor's experiences of learning while studying on their undergraduate programme as introduced to you within scenarios 1 and 2; it is apparent that learning takes place in both the academic and practice setting. Put very simply, learning does not occur in a social vacuum. That is not to say that social factors and media influences completely dictate to you that which you should learn, rather they create a backdrop that pushes you towards particular issues or items of interest (Boronski and Hassan, 2015).

It is arguably important for any healthcare professional to explore what social factors are influencing their learning, but it is perhaps even more important for new graduates transitioning from student to newly registered nurse. As a new member of the profession the need to find your place and fit into the nursing community is strong as you will want to feel a sense of belongingness. This is often coupled with a feeling of uncertainty as you move from the university setting to that of the real world of working as a registered nurse, often within a new team and healthcare organisation. This feeling of uncertainty is discussed in more detail in Chapter 1. Overall, it represents a period in which you as the newly registered nurse can feel vulnerable to outside influences, for better or worse.

Although not a learning theory as such, Lave and Wenger (1991) developed the concept of 'situated learning', a process by which individuals gain entry to what they refer to as a 'community of practice' (Lave and Wenger, 1991). This notion is largely an expansion on the apprenticeship model of learning but it focusses its attention on the social environment in which learning takes place. An important facet of this theory is that the existing members of the community decide on the membership of newcomers. Not necessarily through formal process and procedure, but often informally through the acceptance and approval of the behaviours and values newcomers' exhibit. This is an important distinction since it means that just having the knowledge and skills alone is not enough to enter the community of practice; you need to demonstrate those to the existing members in a way they find acceptable. This in effect is the difference between the 'knowing how' and 'behaving like' of being a nurse. On the one hand, this process is key to ensuring the tacit and unwritten practices and knowledge is passed on to new members, but on the other it promotes the shaping of new members into the image of existing members.

It is quite easy to see how a more junior or student member of staff might want to copy the behaviours and approaches utilised by more experienced or senior colleagues. This may include strategies for promoting exemplary surgical wound care, delegating patient care and communicating with the multi-professional team. At face value it appears that these approaches have worked well for senior colleagues, enabling career progression, so it could be logical to assume that this approach will also work for the more junior member of staff. In most cases this may well be the case, but as systems of healthcare change so too must the behaviours, attitudes and skills of practitioners. The practices adopted by senior colleagues have enabled them to achieve recognition and respect from peers and it is often replication of these acts that drive followership and acceptance of newer and/or junior members of staff. This can, however, present challenges when newer members of staff have different outlooks and views regarding the direction of healthcare provision. In such instances the more senior members of staff are likely to have greater influence over how care is delivered by nature of their experienced status. This can create a tension with newer members of staff who have less influence owing to their lesser experience. Bourdieu explored concepts such as this and coined the term 'symbolic power' (Bourdieu and Passeron, 2000).

As a newly registered nurse, it is very easy to be influenced, often unknowingly, by the expressed (both in action and words) values and behaviours of senior colleagues, particularly those who appear well respected. Similarly, as you progress through your career you will have an increasing number of people using your practice as an example of how they should be behaving. It is in this way that both good and poor practice is spread. Your greatest power in ensuring the delivery of best practice among your peers is through the careful selection of the practice that you choose to adopt.

As you develop and progress throughout your role transition and career it is important that you remain critical in your reflections on your own practice. You will also need to be open to having your own practice challenged and questioned by senior colleagues and more junior members of staff. Not only will this promote a culture of openness, it provides a more critical and questioning approach that can lead to exemplary health-care practice.

Activity 5.5 Critical thinking

Having explored the range of theories, take time to identify how useful each theory could be when applied to your transition from student to registered nurse.

A brief outline answer can be found at the end of this chapter.

Next you will begin to make sense of your learning preferences or learning style and for you to explore the relevance of this information for your transition.

Understanding your learning preferences

You will make sense of your learning preferences through referring back to the two scenarios of Alex a third-year student and Taylor a second-year student and for you to undertake the completion of a learning style questionnaire. This can help you to take a lead on your decision making for learning in transition and throughout your career.

Understanding your learning preferences and the impact of the different theories of learning can support your role transition. A central component of university based education is equipping you with the skills of lifelong learning so that you can continue to learn and grow as your career progresses beyond graduation and towards transition. Being a good learner is not about having the perfect learning technique or approach. A good learner is someone who understands the learning process and their participation in it. In terms of learning preferences this is an understanding of how these preferences impact on your approach and attitude towards learning. Having a low preference for a particular style of learning means you are likely to avoid that approach, and in turn many of the tasks commonly associated with it. If for example you have a low preference for reflective approaches to learning, you may be less likely to engage in reflective discussions about your own practice, which is obviously a concern as a registered nurse. This does not, however, mean that you will never do it, or that you will avoid this at all costs; it just means you are less likely to and may see less value in doing so. Having a firm understanding of your preferences thus enables you to monitor your own actions and behaviours towards learning more closely and look for opportunities to use different approaches to learning.

Activity 5.6   Decision making

Part 1

Reread scenarios 1 and 2 about Alex and Taylor that were first introduced to you at the beginning of this chapter. Both of these scenarios provide information around preferred ways of learning. Once read, make a list of the different learning preferences that you can identify.

A brief outline answer can be found at the end of this chapter.

Part 2

Now, think about your own learning preferences and consider the factors that you feel promote better learning for yourself. Use the list of habits that you identified in Activity 5.3 to inform your answer.

As this part of the activity is based on your own experiences there is no outline answer at the end of the chapter.

In essence what Alex, Taylor and you have described above is your preferred learning style. Kolb (1984) developed a learning styles inventory based on his reflective cycle introduced earlier. While he argued that all four stages of the cycle would need to be completed for learning to take place, he felt that particular individuals had a natural aptitude towards different aspects of the cycle. He named these Divergers, Accommodators, Convergers, and Assimilators.

Honey and Mumford (1992) built upon Kolb's initial work and created a learning style inventory of their own, using the labels Activist, Reflector, Pragmatist and Theorist. Honey and Mumford's inventory is the most often used and this is perhaps due to the more accessible language used and the way that it has been developed into a self-assessment questionnaire. This self-assessment and self-help focus put forward the notion that individuals could use the questionnaire to identify weaker areas in order to develop into a more rounded learner. The electronic link to this and other questionnaires and inventories can be found in the further reading section of the chapter.

Despite widespread use, learning style inventories have received a good degree of criticism. In many instances, there is a degree of questionability in the evidence and research used to develop the tool, as well as the assumptions made in doing so (Coffield, Moseley, Hall and Ecclestone, 2004). There is also criticism relating to the effects of pigeon-holing people over such a tight range and the likelihood of creating self-fulfilling prophecies. This is when a person unknowingly causes a prediction to come true, because it is expected. Despite this learning style, inventories remain very popular and still form a central feature on many courses and programmes that explore learning and teaching.

The important thing to remember when utilising a learning styles inventory, is that it is seeking to highlight a learning preference, not a pre-set thinking mode. This focus on preference for a not fixed style was certainly the intent of Honey and Mumford's work but is often misrepresented. Honey and Mumford sought to provide a language and tool for individuals to think about and thus improve their learning.

Such tools are not hierarchies that suggest that one style or (modality) is superior to others, or that they can be compared between individuals in order to identify the 'better' learner. Instead they should be viewed as tools with which to engage in a reflective dialogue about one's preferences for learning. Take for example Alex and Taylor, introduced to you in scenarios 1 and 2. Provided with the opportunity to complete the Honey and Mumford learning style questionnaire and then discuss the findings with each other, this can help highlight which learning practices Alex and Taylor feel more comfortable with and which might be avoided.

It is not unusual for Alex and Taylor to get an unexpected result, for example Taylor's questionnaire result demonstrates a preference towards the activist learner which is a surprise. This is not to say that the tool is wrong, or that Taylor is wrong. It is instead providing a point for consideration when self-assessing learning practice, and how it may be at odds with how Taylor thinks about learning. Ultimately, identifying your learning 'preference' is about self-exploration and internal critique, not comparison to others or enslavement to one way of thinking or working.

This next activity asks you to undertake a learning styles questionnaire. By doing this you will begin to understand your learning preferences.

Activity 5.7   Evidence based practice and research

There are multiple learning style questionnaires to choose from. The most popular is the Honey and Mumford questionnaire. The further reading section of this chapter provides a sample of questionnaires available. Choose one learning style questionnaire and complete it.

Once you have completed the learning style questionnaire you may wish to reflect on the results with your mentor or personal tutor. As discussed in Chapter 2, using the learning style questionnaire is a form of self-assessment. The evidence can form part of a future SWOT analysis and ultimately part of a subsequent personal development plan. How to develop a personal development plan is discussed in more detail in Chapter 3.

As this activity is based on your own completion of a learning style questionnaire there is no outline answer at the end of the chapter.

> ## Chapter summary
>
> This chapter has helped you to understand how you learn and how this knowledge can be used to support your transition from student to newly registered nurse. You should now have a clearer understanding of how the range of learning theories apply to your transition and your role as a registered nurse. Exploring and understanding your learning preferences is key to identifying your weaknesses as well as the aspects of your development and practice you should focus on to address these. A deeper understanding of the ways in which you learn and the impact your environment and people around you have on that learning is a powerful way to master your own practice. Such awareness will ensure you remain current and up-to-date in your practice and are adaptable for the changings demands of healthcare delivery.

Activities: brief outline answers

Activity 5.1 Reflection (page 100)

Words that you think about when you hear the term 'learning' can be varied and be drawn from personal memories such as a fun activity relating to how you learned to swim. Other words may relate to feelings about joy or disappointment when receiving academic grades.

Key words that may spring to mind will be personal to you and may relate to your capacity to learn at that time, such as 'capacity' and 'challenging'. Words may relate to those relationships that you built while learning, such as 'friendship' and 'sharing ideas with others'.

The words that you have identified could influence your aptitude and confidence for learning.

Activity 5.2 Critical thinking (page 101)

This is an interesting activity as you may never have considered something that you found easy and hard to learn and the factors involved. Some of these factors may be situational, like the time of day, how much sleep you have had, the environment you are in, or when you last ate. Others might be more tied to what it is you are trying to learn. These may include how enjoyable you find it, how well it fits with the knowledge and skills you already have or the way in which you are attempting to learn it. Then there are more human factors that relate to your motivation to learn something and your belief in your ability to succeed in your learning.

Sample of barriers that you may have identified include working shifts while learning and juggling your work–life balance. Others may include grappling with numeracy skills to ensure accurate drug calculation.

Activity 5.3 Decision making (page 101)

Identified below are the possible learning habits reported on by Alex and Taylor that have supported learning (habits with the tick against):

Alex: Motivated to gain new clinical skills; enjoying the formative group presentation; enjoying learning; support from family to study; enjoying developing clinical skills.

Taylor: Learning in small groups and needing time to reflect on information before responding to a question or joining in group work with peers; reading journal papers and critiquing the evidence base; producing mind maps; enjoying online learning and developing clinical skills.

You should have also listed the habits that have supported your learning and it will be interesting to compare and contrast from those identified by Alex and Taylor.

Activity 5.4 Evidence based practice and research (page 102)

You may have applied multiple Internet search engines such as Good Scholar and EBSCO to have found definitions. Further platforms to find research papers includes CINHAL and Medline. An example of a definition of learning is taken from the Oxford English Dictionary; their definition of learning is: *The acquisition of knowledge or skills through study, experience, or being taught.*

Activity 5.5 Critical thinking (page 110)

When thinking about how useful each theory could be when applied to your transition from student to qualified nurse you may have found that you prefer to apply one theory. Alternatively you may have found that there are component parts of each of the theories that you could apply to enhance your future learning. Both of these cases are acceptable.

Behaviourism can help explain how and why different behaviours and practices are adopted by individuals. This theory also extends to being awarded for your behaviours; for example, being thanked by your mentor for the work that you have achieved during a particular shift. Negative reinforcement can be useful as the likelihood of repeating a behaviour/action is increased (reinforced) by the removal of something unpleasant or the avoidance of punishment (negative).

Social learning theory is often a popular learning theory adopted by nurses as the concept of personnel both in the university and clinical learning environment who act as role model can help your journey from student to qualified nurse. It is useful, however, to reflect on what has drawn you to seek a particular role model.

Cognitive learning theory involves reflecting on past experiences and using mental models to explore different ideas and options. As nurses, this model can be particularly useful for role transition as it helps to build a mental picture of 'what if' scenarios that may or may not have yet occurred or have been experienced before.

Social aspects of learning: an example of how social aspects of learning could be applied to your transition from student to qualified nurse is through adopting an open mind and a culture of critical enquiry and exploration. Consider the placement of power and influence.

Activity 5.6 Decision making (page 111)

From the scenarios you may have identified the following learning preferences: learn in small groups; time to reflect on information before responding to a question or joining in group work with peers; enjoys reading journal papers and critiquing the evidence base; producing mind maps; online learning.

Further reading

Benedict, C (2015) *How We Learn: The surprising truth about when, where, and why it happens.* London: Random House.

This is an easy to read and contemporary book with very clear examples of real world application of learning theory.

Knowles, MS, Holton, EF and Swanson, RA (2014) *The Adult Learner* (8th edn). London and New York: Routledge.

This builds upon Knowles earlier work that explores learning adulthood with a particular focus on learning for success in the workplace.

Useful websites

There are a good number of different learning styles inventories and questionnaires, and links to some of the more common ones are given below. As noted above, remember to use these with caution; when used responsibly they can be very powerful in understanding your learning, used incorrectly and they will limit you.

The VARK questionnaire

http://vark-learn.com/the-vark-questionnaire/

http://vark-learn.com/
The Honey and Mumford questionnaire

http://resources.eln.io/honey-mumford-learner-types-1986-questionnaire-online/

Chapter 6

Identifying and developing clinical leadership in relation to transition

Angelina Chadwick and Jacqueline Leigh

NMC Standards for Pre-registration Nursing Education

This chapter will address the following competencies:

Domain 4: Leadership, management and team working

Generic competences

- All nurses must be professionally accountable and use clinical governance processes to maintain and improve nursing practice and standards of healthcare. They must be able to respond autonomously and confidently to planned and uncertain situations, managing themselves and others effectively. They must create and maximise opportunities to improve services. They must also demonstrate the potential to develop further management and leadership skills during their period of preceptorship and beyond.

Competencies

1. All nurses must act as change agents and provide leadership through quality improvement and service development to enhance people's wellbeing and experiences of healthcare.
2. All nurses must systematically evaluate care and ensure that they and others use the findings to help improve people's experience and care outcomes and to shape future services.
3. All nurses must be able to identify priorities and manage time and resources effectively to ensure the quality of care is maintained or enhanced.
4. All nurses must be self-aware and recognise how their own values, principles and assumptions may affect their practice. They must maintain their own personal and professional development, learning from experience, through supervision, feedback, reflection and evaluation.

5.   All nurses must facilitate nursing students and others to develop their competence, using a range of professional and personal development skills.

6.   All nurses must work independently as well as in teams. They must be able to take the lead in coordinating, delegating and supervising care safely, managing risk and remaining accountable for the care given.

7.   All nurses must work effectively across professional and agency boundaries, actively involving and respecting others' contributions to integrated person-centred care. They must know when and how to communicate with and refer to other professionals and agencies in order to respect the choices of service users and others, promoting shared decision making, to deliver positive outcomes and to coordinate smooth, effective transition within and between services and agencies.

Essential Skills Clusters

This chapter will address the following ESCs:

Cluster: Care, compassion and communication

1.   As partners in the care process, people can trust a newly registered graduate nurse to provide collaborative care based on the highest standards, knowledge and competence.

1.8.   Demonstrates clinical confidence through sound knowledge, skills and understanding relevant to field.

1.9.   Is self-aware and self-confident, knows own limitations and is able to take appropriate action.

1.10.   Acts as a role model in promoting a professional image.

1.11.   Acts as a role model in developing trusting relationships, within professional boundaries.

5.   People can trust the newly registered graduate nurse to engage with them in a warm, sensitive and compassionate way.

5.10.   Has insight into own values and how these may impact on interactions with others.

Cluster: Organisational aspects of care

9.   People can trust the newly registered graduate nurse to treat them as partners and work with them to make a holistic and systematic assessment of their

(Continued)

(Continued)

needs; to develop a personalised plan that is based on mutual understanding and respect for their individual situation, promoting health and well-being, minimising risk of harm and promoting their safety at all times.

9.14.   Applies research based evidence to practice.

12.   People can trust the newly registered graduate nurse to respond to their feedback and a wide range of other sources to learn, develop and improve services.

12.6.   Actively responds to feedback.

14.   People can trust the newly registered graduate nurse to be an autonomous and confident member of the multi-disciplinary or multi agency team and to inspire confidence in others.

14.8.   Takes effective role within the team adopting the leadership role when appropriate.

14.9.   Acts as an effective role model in decision making, taking action and supporting others.

14.10. Works inter-professionally and autonomously as a means of achieving optimum outcomes for people.

16.   People can trust the newly registered graduate nurse to safely lead, co-ordinate and manage care.

16.1.   Inspires confidence and provides clear direction to others.

16.2.   Takes decisions and is able to answer for these decisions when required.

16.3.   Bases decisions on evidence and uses experience to guide decision-making.

16.4.   Acts as a positive role model for others.

16.5.   Manages time effectively.

16.6.   Negotiates with others in relation to balancing competing and conflicting priorities.

Chapter aims

After reading this chapter you will be able to:

- describe the differences between leadership and management and their relevance to transition;
- examine what is meant by clinical leadership;
- explore the NHS Healthcare Leadership Model, and other self-assessment tools that help promote effective leadership development;
- undertake a SWOT analysis to provide a visual map of the information generated from the self-assessment;
- create a transition focused person development plan (PDP) based on the content of the self-assessment and SWOT analysis.

Introduction

This chapter will explore the concepts of leadership and management. This chapter will first define leadership and management and then discuss what is meant by clinical leadership. Next, self-assessment will be applied to help determine areas of leadership strength and to identify weaknesses or areas for leadership development. A SWOT analysis is used to make sense of the information generated through undertaking the self-assessments. Finally, all of the information generated is focussed upon to develop individual TFPDPs. Activities throughout this chapter that include being introduced to a case study about Sam, provide the opportunity to reflect, plan and develop the leadership required for transition. These leadership skills enable high quality care that takes place within an ever-changing healthcare environment.

What is leadership?

Before starting this section, Activity 6.1 asks you to reflect upon your own knowledge around what is leadership.

Activity 6.1   Reflection

Spend a few moments thinking about leadership. What does the term mean to you and your transition? Can you think of any examples where you have had to demonstrate your leadership skills?

A brief outline answer can be found at the end of this chapter.

Leadership is multifaceted with many definitions and qualities. Leadership can be misunderstood by nurses who perceive it as something that only applies to senior managers or to those leading the organisation. So what is leadership? A plethora of definitions exist for leadership both within and outside of the healthcare arena. While there is no single agreed definition among researchers and writers, there are some fundamental elements that need to be considered and these include: the ability to influence others, have followers and common goals. A simple definition involves one person influencing others, but this relationship needs to be driven by a clear vision or shared purpose to achieve a common goal. Leaders should support and motivate others to act and achieve mutually agreed goals. Therefore, for the purpose of this chapter, leadership is defined as influencing and motivating others to work effectively to meet the goals and objectives of the service and the wider organisation. Leadership may be formal, where it is linked to one's role and hierarchy but it may also be informal when leadership skills are used to influence without formal role recognition.

Having considered some definitions of leadership the dimension of clinical leadership needs to be explored next. Clinical leadership can be defined as providing excellent patient and client care through undertaking service improvement. Dimensions include promoting the values of the NHS through inspiring, motivating and empowering others to meet the needs of the patient or client. In other words, Leigh, Williamson and Rutherford (2017) suggest that clinical leadership is a key part of every nurse or clinician's role, whereby they have a responsibility to contribute to the provision of an effective service and shape its future direction. An example of this would be where a newly registered nurse contributes ideas and suggestions to improve a service area in order to deliver high quality patient care. This could be through a change in process, highlighting the service limitations or suggesting new ways of working to the ward/ team manager. This would demonstrate responsiveness to addressing patients' needs and reporting of any issues that may prohibit. Throughout this chapter the term leadership will be used to also encompass clinical leadership.

A fundamental component of effective leadership is the ability to manage oneself. Needed is an ability to recognise our personal qualities and behaviours. These include self-awareness, self-confidence, self-knowledge, personal reflection, resilience and determination. Debated are the key attributes required to be an effective leader and these include clarity, integrity, courage, trust, humility, compassion and vulnerability. The Francis Report (2013) outlines qualities that include some of the attributes discussed above that are required of leaders at all levels of healthcare service. Table 6.1 below illustrates some of the common leadership qualities found in the literature with examples relating to clinical practice.

Leadership quality	Examples in clinical practice
Ability to create and communicate vision and strategy	As a registered nurse to be able to explain to a student, new staff member or patient the overarching aims of the service area/ward. To be able to effectively communicate any changes to approaches to care, patient pathways and ways of working effectively.
Understanding of how to prioritise and protect safety and provision of fundamental standards within available services	A registered nurse understands and is able to demonstrate the effective prioritisation of patient care while adhering to organisational policies and procedures.
Ability to be viewed as a role model	Being a role model to learners in the placement area as in exemplifying the roles and responsibilities of a professionally registered nurse. To be a role model for other members of the nursing profession and to patients in terms of upholding and adhering to professional, organisational and national standards.

Leadership quality	Examples in clinical practice
Listening and learning from patients and colleagues	As a registered nurse taking time to elicit feedback and listen to patients, colleagues and members of the wider multi-professional team. This includes suggestions, opinions and constructive criticism to improve the service in order to be able to provide high quality patient care.
Inspirational and motivating colleagues	To be innovative and suggest new ideas/ways of working in practice. To encourage and support colleagues when they have ideas and suggestions to enhance the patient/learner/team experience in their service.
Willingness to challenge	To have the courage to say when you think something is wrong to those around you, including decision makers. This may include challenging colleagues with regards to their practice. To be able to question treatment pathways for patients in your care when new evidence is available suggesting alternatives.
Ability to judge and analyse complex issues	As a registered nurse being able to review information, this may be feedback from stakeholders/patients, and analyse issues. Alternatively responding to a patient's complex care needs or changes in physiological observations. Analysing the information to hand, being able to respond and manage in a timely manner.
Probity	As a registered nurse the quality of having strong moral principles (probity) is requisite of the NMC Code of Conduct (2015). Honesty in all interactions and behaviour is crucial to nursing practice. Informing patients when they have a long wait in the Emergency department, breaking of bad news, explaining interventions/treatments in an open and honest manner even when they may be unpalatable for the patient.
Openness	To be open and transparent wherever possible in all interactions and communications with learners, colleagues, patients and carers.
Courage	As a registered nurse to have the courage to question those in senior positions, to challenge poor practice to protect the patient and those within the service. To whistle blow and raise concerns to senior managers.

Table 6.1 Leadership qualities

Having explored some of the common leadership qualities found in the literature it is important to know that leadership is not a new concept. There are many theories and approaches that are explored in some books listed in the further reading section of this chapter. It is, however, generally accepted that leadership skills, qualities and behaviours can be developed through education and while engaging in clinical practice. Ways for nurses in role transition to advance clinical leadership development is examined later in this chapter.

Exploring the differences between leadership and management

Leadership occurs in groups where people work towards a mutual purpose; however leadership also requires considerable management skills. This indicates that leadership and management are inextricably linked. Management includes planning, budgeting, organising, staffing, controlling and problem solving. Leadership involves establishing direction, aligning people, motivating and inspiring. Leadership and management strive to achieve the same but use different approaches. Northouse (2015) further outlines the differences between leadership and management (see Table 6.2) and concludes that management is about function and leadership is about movement. Northouse also suggests that management and leadership development is not simply about acquiring management skills but the development of approaches for effective leadership.

Management	Leadership
Planning and budgeting	Establishing direction
Establishing agendas	Creating a vision
Setting timetables	Clarifying the big picture
Allocating resources	Setting strategies
Organizing and staffing	Aligning people
Providing structure	Communicating goals
Making job placements	Seeking commitment
Establishing rules and procedures	Building teams and coalitions
Controlling and problem solving	Motivating and inspiring
Developing incentives	Inspiring and energising
Generating creative solutions	Empowering subordinates
Taking corrective action	Satisfying unmet needs

Table 6.2 Management versus leadership

Having identified the differences between management and leadership, an applied example relating to the newly registered nurse is provided next.

The management behaviour of controlling and problem solving may be seen when a student nurse or staff member approaches a newly registered nurse with a patient issue relating to the management of the patient discharge. Here the newly registered nurse takes control of the situation by taking over and coordinating the patient discharge, thus personally dealing with the issue. Whereas when adopting motivating and inspiring behaviours the newly registered nurse who is approached by the same student or staff member with the same patient discharge issue would encourage the staff member to consider options themselves, maybe even suggest ideas, but encourage the staff member to work through the issue with support and not take over. This illustrates the managing behaviours of 'doing things right' and leading by 'doing the right things'.

As a student nurse you need to consider the management responsibilities and functions of your role. It is important to remember that management is a vital element of leadership development.

Self-assessing your leadership – the NHS Healthcare Leadership Model and other tools

Self-assessment is an important part of your role transition. As a student you should use self-assessment to understand the leadership and management skills, behaviours and attributes that you already possess. Reflection is an important part of the self-assessment process. Self-assessment has been discussed within Chapter 2 and reflection in Chapter 3. When contemplating leadership development you can use one of the many leadership assessment tools to help you. The NHS Healthcare Leadership Model (NHS Leadership Academy, 2013) is one of the most recently developed tools and comprises nine 'leadership dimensions' of leadership behaviour (Table 6.3). Read the table and look at the examples provided linking the leadership dimensions to your role transition.

The Healthcare Leadership Model was devised for all healthcare practitioners, even those without formal leadership responsibilities. It was designed to be an evolving model, meaning that it will change over time in line with healthcare service changes. It suggests that leadership behaviours exhibited by people can affect the culture and climate of the service. Also, what you do and the way you behave can impinge on the patients' experience and on the quality of service provided. Each of the nine dimensions exemplifies desired leadership behaviours. These behaviours are ranked using a four-part scale, from 'Essential; Proficient; Strong to Exemplary'. While the complexity of these behaviours increases through the scale these are not related to job roles or hierarchies. All nine dimensions of the model are important to an individual's leadership development. The model has been designed to guide practitioners to identify where individual leadership strengths lie and areas for future development. Self-assessments can be undertaken by registering online at www.leadershipacademy. nhs.uk/resources/healthcare-leadership-model/ and completing the questionnaire. The self-assessment comprises statements around each of the behaviours relating to each dimension and requires the individual to self-rate and score each one.

There are other leadership development self-assessment tools and these include the leadership, management and team working (Domain 4) generic and/or field

Leadership dimension	What does it mean for student nurses in role transition?
Inspiring shared purpose	As a student nurse you need to behave in a way that reflects the principles and values of the NHS. Are you a role model for others? Do you understand that what you do affects patient care?
Leading with care	Having the essential personal qualities to lead and care for the needs of the team. As a student nurse do you notice upset team members? Do you try and support them?
Evaluating information	Seeking information and using it to develop innovatively, making evidence based decisions for all concerned. Do you gather feedback from patients? Do you consider the impact of feedback on improving service provision?
Connecting our service	Understanding the healthcare service arena and the connectedness. Do you know how the service area (ward/placement area) works with other service areas? Do you understand how services work together and why?
Sharing the vision	Communicating the vision with motivation. Can you communicate honestly, appropriately at the right time to people at the right levels?
Engaging the team	Involving individuals and valuing their contributions for improvements. Within a ward team/service do you listen and value team member's views and suggestions?
Holding to account	Clear goals and direction to support individuals to take responsibility and provide feedback. Do you take responsibility for your own performance? Do you self-assess and set SMART goals to work towards?
Developing capability	Developing oneself and others using a variety of methods to ensure future needs are met. Do you look for opportunities to develop yourself? Do you support others to develop?
Influencing for results	Having a positive impact on others and developing relationships to build collaboration. Do you express your views clearly? Can you present clear arguments?

Table 6.3 The Healthcare Leadership Model

specific competencies within the Nursing and Midwifery Council (NMC) Standards for Pre-registration Education (NMC, 2010). At the beginning of this chapter generic leadership, management and team working competencies were listed. You may want to explore some of the more field specific ones as part of your self-assessment. These can be found online at the NMC website.

As you start your career as a professional nurse you can use the competencies listed in the standards for pre-registration to guide you through the process of self-assessment. This can be done for every generic and field specific competence. As part of the self-assessment process you need to generate the evidence of why you feel that you have certain leadership strengths or whether you are beginning to identify any weaknesses. Types of evidence you should consider include: feedback from mentors, personal tutors, patients/service users/carers, reflective pieces and assessment feedback. Evidence may also be generated through undertaking other self-assessments. These may include the Key Skills (Dearing, 1997) or Johari Window. The weaknesses will be your areas of development that you need to improve and develop.

This next activity provides you with an opportunity to critically think about self-assessment.

Activity 6.2   Critical thinking

Read the first generic leadership and management competence below. Consider your evidence and feedback from practice: is this an area of strength or weakness? Assign a number or colour to the competence below to indicate an area of strength or weakness.

1.   All nurses must act as change agents and provide leadership through quality improvement and service development to enhance people's wellbeing and experiences of healthcare.

Do you feel you can act as a change agent? Have you undertaken or been involved in change to enhance service development? If so, where is your evidence to support this? Mark it in the colour green for yes or assign a score of 1 to it. If not, then mark it in red or assign it a score of 3. If you are unsure, then mark it in yellow and score it a 2. If this competence is marked in green or assigned a low score this will indicate an area of strength. If highlighted in yellow, red or assigned a higher score then this is an area of weakness that should be developed into a TFPDP.

As this activity is based on your own experiences there is no outline answer at the end of the chapter.

Using the same approach as discussed above, a job description can also be used as a self-assessment tool. A job description can be defined as a high level statement of those tasks and duties an individual should perform. All jobs should have job descriptions or role outlines that an employee will work to. Potential job applicants can refer to this when considering suitability for a post. Leadership and management skills will be identified in most job descriptions; however, these will differ dependent upon the level of the position it relates to. To self-assess against a job description you will first need to find a suitable job description for a post you are interested in applying for when you qualify. Read the job summary and then the main duties and responsibilities in relation to leadership and management for the post. Then using the self-assessment methods discussed above, identify your areas of strength and those for development. Once you have identified your weaknesses from the main duties and responsibilities within the job description then you can develop a PDP around these.

An example below is taken from a band 5 job description for a staff nurse post in a children and adolescent mental health service (CAMHS) inpatient unit. In the job summary the following statement is written that relates to leadership and management:

> *You will be responsible for the assessment, planning, implementation and evaluation of programmes of care for young people with serious mental health issues and/or complex emotional/behavioural difficulties. This will be in conjunction with the multi-disciplinary team.*
>
> *You will supervise the work of junior staff, ensuring the highest possible standard of care in accordance with policies, procedures and legislation.*
>
> *You will participate in clinical supervision and have an active role in the development of the multi-disciplinary team. This includes participation in the education programmes of students and others.*

Reading the expectations of the band 5 post above, the job summary illustrates elements of management and leadership. You need to ask yourself the following: Have you assessed, planned, implemented and evaluated a programme of care? Have you supervised junior staff? Have you had an active role in the development of the multi-disciplinary team? All these areas require management and leadership knowledge and skills, which you could be expected to demonstrate if you were thinking of applying for this post.

NHS Knowledge and Skills Framework

Following the theme of competencies and role responsibilities we will now discuss NHS Knowledge and Skills Framework (KSF) (DoH, 2004). The NHS developed the KSF as a development framework to aid staff in career and pay progression. It describes the knowledge and skills that NHS staff need to apply in their work in order to deliver quality services. The KSF is made up of 30 dimensions (Table 6.4).

There are six core dimensions that apply to every NHS role. The remaining 24 are called specific dimensions, some of which apply to some jobs but not all. Each dimension is made up of four levels that are role and level defined. Each level has a title called a level descriptor, which describes what it is about. Attached to these descriptors are indicators that describe the knowledge and skills needed for the levels. Leadership, management and team working knowledge and skills are implicit within the higher levels of these dimensions. Therefore, this framework can be used as a self-assessment tool when considering your role transition. The ideal place to start with this framework would be the six core dimensions. It is advised that you read each level descriptor and indicator (see an example of one below) and then undertake the self-assessment. Those areas highlighted for development should then be transferred to a TFPDP.

Core dimensions (6)	Specific dimensions (24)
1 Communication	HW1–10 Health and wellbeing
2 Personal and people development	EF1–3 Estates and facilities
3 Health safety and security	IK1–3 Information and knowledge
4 Service improvement	G1–8 General
5 Quality	
6 Equality and diversity	

Table 6.4   The NHS Knowledge and Skills Framework

Having viewed the KSF dimensions in Table 6.4 you will next find an example of a level descriptor followed by an indicator relating to core dimension one – Communication.

Core dimension 1 level 1: Communicate with a limited range of people on day-to-day matters

Indicator

The worker: communicates with a limited range of people on a day-to-day matter in a form that is appropriate to the situation.

For more information relating to the KSF please refer to the document link at the end of this chapter.

Next you are introduced to a case study about Sam who is a third year student nurse. This case study will help you to further apply the concepts of leadership and management to your role transition particularly when exploring self-assessment, SWOT and SNOB analysis and personal development planning.

Scenario: Sam

Sam is an undergraduate student nurse (mental health field) who is entering the third and final year of the programme and has undertaken all placements at a Mental Health NHS Foundation Trust within the North of England. Practice placements have included an acute ward, a community mental health team, a child and adolescent mental health service (CAMHS) and adult RAID (risks, assumptions, issues and dependencies). RAID is a service that provides a rapid response to people attending

(Continued)

(Continued)

the emergency department and urgent care centre to offer a mental health need and risk assessment. Sam has two further practice placements to undertake before qualifying as a registered mental health nurse.

Feedback from clinical mentors has indicated good team working and communication skills with a need to delegate to healthcare assistants and others. Sam also recognises inexperience when taking the lead in multidisciplinary team (MDT) meetings.

While on the acute ward placement, Sam has been provided with opportunities to work with the Quality Improvement Lead within the Trust. Sam is now much more aware of the mission of the Trust and some of the service objectives. Sam has passed all academic components of the nursing programme so far and likes to teach when in practice and has received positive feedback from patients and other students regarding teaching ability. Sam has engaged with personal development planning since the first year of the programme and is developing an ability to set SMART goals.

Sam is about to embark on a preparation for a role transition module but does not really understand what transition entails. This is something that has not really been considered yet.

Al, a newly registered staff nurse in the current placement, has discussed personal experience of role transition. Recalling feeling nervous and excited at the same time, Al has suggested that Sam should take responsibility as a third year student nurse and undertake some self-assessments and personal development planning in relation to leadership and management. Sam identifies lack of knowledge around systems for feedback.

This next activity provides a further opportunity to practice your skills of self-assessment through using the case study of Sam introduced to you.

Activity 6.3   Leadership and management

Self-assessment – Considering the case study of Sam, undertake a leadership focussed self-assessment as if you were Sam. Using the NMC pre-registration generic or field specific standard competencies relating to domain 4 – leadership, management and team working, identify three potential key areas of leadership development for Sam. These potential key areas may include Sam's abilities to: act as change agent and provide leadership through quality improvement and service development to enhance people's wellbeing and experience of healthcare; prioritise and manage time and resources effectively to ensure the quality of care is maintained; and work independently as well as in teams.

A brief outline answer of this part of the activity can be found at the end of this chapter.

Now that you have applied the self-assessment tool to Sam, take some time to consider choosing one self-assessment tool and apply to your own personal transition, specifically focussing on your leadership and management development needs. An example of a self-assessment tool that you could choose is the NMC pre-registration competencies, in particular domain 4 – leadership, management and team working generic and/or field specific standard competencies. Another includes use of the qualified nurse job description. Try to identify three areas for your own leadership development.

As this part of the activity is based on your own experiences there is no outline answer at the end of the chapter.

Now that you have undertaken the self-assessment it is important to make sense of the information generated and this can be achieved through undertaking a SWOT or SNOB analysis.

SWOT or SNOB analysis

Chapter 2 introduced you to the concept of a SWOT and SNOB analysis. Application of either of these tools will provide you with a clear analysis of your current leadership development needs based on information generated through undertaking the self-assessment. When undertaking a SWOT or SNOB analysis, strengths in relation to leadership and role transition may include an ability to apply quality improvement tools to measure patient outcomes. A weakness may include mentor feedback around insufficient delegation skills. A need may include support from the mentor to develop skills for delegation. Opportunities may relate to shadowing service improvement leads in the hospital and participating in service improvement projects. Threats may relate to personal confidence with managing resources or participating in a nurse led patient handover. Finally, barriers may include lack of confidence when managing risk.

The next activity provides you with the opportunity to practise using the SWOT tool through its application to the case study about Sam the third year student nurse.

In Chapter 3 you have been introduced to the concept of TFPDP and the setting of SMART short- and long-term goals. The benefits of producing TFPDPs include providing you with a mechanism to take ownership of your own learning, identify learning opportunities and verify your achievements during the transition journey. Development of SMART leadership focussed goals will ensure that each of your goals is specific, making

Activity 6.4 Decision making

Undertake a SWOT analysis based on the information generated from undertaking the leadership and management focussed self-assessment on Sam (Activity 6.3). This will enable you to generate a visual picture of the information produced that can then be transferred to the TFPDP.

A brief outline answer can be found at the end of this chapter.

them easily manageable and achievable. Goals that are measurable means that your leadership achievements can be verified by others such as preceptor and mentor. Setting small, achievable and realistic targets that together build towards the final goal will help you to gain confidence as you progress through your transition. Goals that are timely support role transition because they provide the timeline to work towards and help you manage resources.

The next part of this chapter builds on this information and provides the opportunity to generate a TFPDP specifically for your leadership development. Having explored and identified your own self-assessed areas and undertaken a SWOT analysis you can now develop each of your weaknesses into individual TFPDPs.

TFPDP – leadership specific

In order to develop a TFPDP it must start with an identified need. For Sam one of the identified needs is being able to delegate patient care to members of the nursing team. This is in line with generic competence 6 taken from domain 4 of the NMC standards for pre-registration education. SMART short- and long-term goals will need to be developed.

In order to be able to help Sam develop and meet these goals some resources will need to be identified. The success criteria within the TFPDP will identify how you know when you have achieved your planned goals. In Sam's example the achievement of delegation will include assessment and feedback by the mentor. This is evidenced by the signing off by the mentor of relevant NMC competences within Sam's practice placement documentation. A review date must always be included in order to keep the TFPDPs timely in practice.

This next activity will provide you with the opportunity to write a leadership development focussed PDP for Sam.

It would now be useful for you to develop your own three TFPDPs in relation to your identified areas of weakness found within your SWOT analysis.

Activity 6.5   Problem solving

As Sam, develop three PDPs based on the weaknesses identified within the SWOT analysis. You may wish to use a colour or number coded system to relate to each of the TFPDPs required. For example, Sam's academic need could be in green or assign a number one, professional need in orange, number two, with the academic area of development in blue or number 3. Remember to apply the SMART framework so that each is manageable and achievable.

A brief outline answer can be found at the end of this chapter.

Chapter summary

This chapter has defined and explored the concepts of leadership and management and clinical leadership. Self-assessment around these areas in relation to the NMC standards for pre-registration education has been discussed together with examples of other leadership and management self-assessment frameworks. A case study has been used to provide examples of a self-assessment in the areas of leadership and management development. The SWOT analysis has been used to make sense of the information generated from the self-assessments. Finally, TFPDPs have been developed based on the weaknesses identified from the SWOT analysis and used to formulate leadership and management specific goals and actions.

Activities: brief outline answers

Activity 6.1 Reflection (page 119)

What is leadership?

You will have found that there are many definitions for leadership. There is no right or wrong definition of leadership. The key message is for you to choose one that fits with your own values. Clinical leadership is unique to healthcare because it has the patient at the forefront. It is important to remember that effective leadership requires you to manage yourself. It is how you influence others that has the greatest impact on delivering excellent nursing care.

Activity 6.3 Leadership and management (page 128)

Self-assessment

Undertake a self-assessment as Sam using the NMC pre-registration generic competencies and identify three key areas of leadership development for Sam.

You have undertaken a self-assessment, as Sam, using the NMC standards for pre-registration education in particular domain 4 relating to leadership, management and team working.

Sam has identified the following areas to develop in. Sam has spent some time with the quality improvement lead but feels that this is an area that needs to be developed further. Feedback from mentors has indicated a need to delegate to healthcare assistants and others; Sam also recognises the need to take the lead in MDT meetings to support quality patient care and develop leadership skills.

Activity 6.4 Decision making (page 130)

SWOT analysis

Provided is an example of a SWOT analysis for Sam based on the results from the leadership-focussed self-assessment.

Strengths	Weaknesses
1. Spent time with quality improvement lead, recognise need to improve quality in care 2. Feedback from mentors includes good team worker and good communication skills 3. Good communication skills with service users	1. Need to develop an awareness of mechanisms for feedback in order to improve quality in care 2. Need to be able to delegate to nursing team 3. To advocate for patients and take the lead in multidisciplinary ward meetings
Opportunities	**Threats**
1. Discuss with mentors in placement 2. Two placement areas available to undertake delegation 3. Have a ward placement option available	1. Lack of knowledge around systems for feedback 2. Lack of confidence and knowledge to be able to delegate 3. The knowledge to be able to competently lead and present in the MDT

Table 6.5 Example SWOT analysis activity

Activity 6.5 Problem solving (page 131)

This activity required you to write a TFPDP (leadership specific).

An example of SMART goals relating to Sam's leadership focussed professional development needs are:

* *short-term goal: to be able to competently delegate the care for four patients to the nursing team during four shifts, in first placement in the final year of programme under the supervision of a mentor;*
* *long-term goal: to be able to delegate all the care of a ward of patients to the nursing team over a whole shift on a weekly basis by the end of the final placement of programme under the supervision of a mentor.*

Resources for this particular TFPDP will include reading some nursing leadership and management textbooks and journals. An example would be The Royal College of Nursing (RCN) who has produced guidance on delegation. Sam would need to shadow and observe mentors and qualified nurses in practice delegating to the wider team. A discussion about delegation with nursing staff and the wider team would be required. Finally Sam would need the opportunity to practise the skills and to be given feedback on her effectiveness.

Further reading

Ellis, P and Bach, S (2015) *Leadership, Management and Team Working in Nursing* (2nd edn). London: Learning Matters, SAGE.

This textbook is comprehensive in its content around leadership and management issues within healthcare.

Sullivan, EJ and Garland, G (2013) *Practical Leadership and Management in Nursing* (2nd edn). Harlow, UK: Pearson Education.

Practical Leadership is a useful textbook since it is aimed at a UK audience and is focussed around the NHS. It is also a useful practical leadership and management guide that is very readable.

Journals

The journals listed below are all useful resources in terms of leadership and management issues related to nursing and healthcare.

- *Journal of Nursing Management* – this is an international research based nursing management journal. It seeks to build on management and leadership knowledge for practitioners, academics, policymakers and managers.
- *Nursing Management* – an RCN produced journal, aimed at current and aspiring nurse leaders, providing research, clinical and continuing professional development management articles.
- *Nurse Leader* – a practical and skills based, easy to read journal aimed at current and aspiring nurse leaders.

Useful websites

www.leadershipacademy.nhs.uk/resources/healthcare-leadership-model/

The leadership academy hosts most of the information relating to healthcare leadership as well as the healthcare leadership model. This body promote their leadership development programmes designed for staff at many different levels.

www.kingsfund.org.uk/leadership

The Kings Fund is an independent body that undertakes research in many health-related areas. They have a dedicated section on their website to healthcare leadership and management. They also advise the Department of Health on health-related policy matters. You can sign up for their free weekly newsletter.

www.rcn.org.uk/professional-development/accountability-and-delegation

This RCN guide has been developed solely around accountability and delegation issues and may be useful if you wish to develop in this area.

Chapter 7 Transition support

Chris Fisher and Melanie Stephens

NMC Standards for Pre-registration Nursing Education

This chapter addresses the following competencies:

Domain 1: Professional values

Competencies:

7. All nurses must be responsible and accountable for keeping their knowledge and skills up to date through continuing professional development. They must aim to improve their performance and enhance the safety and quality of care through evaluation, supervision and appraisal.
8. All nurses must practice independently, recognising the limits of their competence and knowledge. They must reflect on these limits and seek advice from, or refer to, other professionals where necessary.

Domain 4: Leadership, management and team working

Competencies:

4. All nurses must be self-aware and recognise how their own values, principles and assumptions may affect their practice. They must maintain their own personal and professional development, learning from experience, through supervision, feedback, reflection and evaluation.
6. All nurses must work independently as well as in teams. They must be able to take the lead in co-ordinating, delegating and supervising care safely, managing risk and remaining accountable for the care given.

Essential Skills Clusters

This chapter will address the following ESCs:

Progression point:

1.2. Works within the limitations of the role and recognises level of competence.

1.7. Uses professional support structures to learn from experience and make appropriate adjustments.

1.9. Is self-aware and self-confident, knows own limitations and is able to take appropriate action.

1.14. Uses professional support structures to develop self-awareness, challenge own prejudices and enable professional relationships, so that care is delivered without compromise.

Progression point:

12.3. Uses supervision and other forms of reflective learning to make effective use of feedback.

12.4. Takes feedback from colleagues, managers and other departments seriously and shares the messages with others and members of the team.

12.6. Actively responds to feedback.

12.8. As an individual team member and team leader, actively seeks and learns from feedback to enhance care and own and others' professional development.

Chapter aims

After reading this chapter you will be able to:

- describe the roles and responsibilities of preceptors and preceptees and identify similarities and differences between mentoring, preceptorship and clinical supervision;
- appreciate the importance of seeking out and being receptive to constructive feedback as a newly registered nurse;
- identify other networks and resources that can assist with transition support;
- understand why it is your duty to always work within the limits of your knowledge and clinical competence.

Introduction

The purpose of this chapter is to recognise and understand the importance of support to develop into an autonomous practitioner during your transition from student nurse to newly registered nurse. This chapter will help you to identify what support systems are currently available and how this can affect your job performance. The chapter will also help you to identify when and how you should commence clinical decision making in order to develop your autonomy. The chapter will begin by introducing you to imposter syndrome and the impact this can have on your transition. It then moves on to explore transition support and how this will change from mentorship to preceptorship or another form. You will then have an opportunity to explore what supernumerary status means as a newly registered nurse and how feedback should be provided. Finally, the chapter will identify what other forms of support are available and how this will help you to develop your autonomy and clinical decision-making skills.

Scenario: Marek

Marek is a newly registered nurse who obtained a first staff nurse post in a local NHS Trust. Marek was appointed to a preceptor, Gayle, on the first week of employment.

Although Marek felt competent and knowledgeable as a third-year student, the position of a registered nurse with the increased responsibility and accountability led to feelings of self-doubt and low confidence.

On commencing employment Marek found that Gayle and the other staff appeared too busy to help answer any questions raised. As time passed Marek became increasingly anxious and did not fully understand the role of the staff nurse and what was expected. This led to feelings of being an imposter. This job did not match expectations and Marek began to have sleepless nights, phoned in sick and started to consider whether this was the right profession.

Finally, Marek decided to approach Gayle, an experienced registered nurse, to express these concerns. Gayle was surprised and had thought that Marek was coping. Once this misunderstanding was addressed, although Gayle was often busy with workload responsibilities, Marek's questions were always answered, and time was made to discuss caseload and offer guidance. Gayle would often work alongside Marek and offer feedback, encouragement and support on any progress, this helped to improve Marek's confidence.

Marek discovered that the Trust also offered occasional study days for newly registered nurses. When attending study days Marek developed existing skills as well as skills required of a registered nurse. Marek met with other newly registered nurses, shared stories, experiences and gained valuable support.

This scenario is intended to highlight the potential for newly registered nurses to leave the profession due to their expectations not matching experiences in practice and the lack of personal resilience and coping strategies; this is demonstrated in figures collated by the NMC where during 2016–17 more than 29,000 registered nurses allowed their registration to lapse.

This chapter aims to help you to identify and utilise the support and resources that will be available to you when you make the transition from student to newly registered nurse, and to recognise some of the potential problems that you may face. It is anticipated that once you are familiar with the concept of preceptorship, the role of your preceptor/support person and your own responsibilities as a preceptee/newly registered nurse you will be able to build your own network of support, advice and feedback in your chosen clinical area.

Imposter syndrome and transition

It may seem surprising that many high achieving individuals feel like a fraud when they first register as a professional and take up their first post. They think they haven't the skills and knowledge others believe they have. Feeling like this is more common than you think and most people at some point in their life will feel like a phoney. However, when feeling like a fraud gets out of control it can develop into something called imposter syndrome (Kearns, 2016) and this can affect how you think and behave.

Imagine what it will be like on your first day as a newly registered nurse in your first post, wearing the uniform of a newly registered nurse. You are charged with the responsibilities that come with the role and no doubt you will have had both positive and negative feelings; being a newly registered nurse can be both exciting and unnerving.

Don't worry you are not alone!

As you have read in Chapter 1, the transition that student nurses go through to becoming newly registered nurses can be both exciting and stressful. Kramer (1974) described how newly registered nurses experienced 'reality shock'. This reality shock occurs with the transition from education to the clinical setting where there are different priorities and pressures. Seminal research by Duchscher (2009) referred to the 'transition shock' that nurses experience as they realise that they are professionally accountable for their actions and need to rapidly become acquainted with increased autonomy and local responsibilities.

Indeed, the transitional experiences of newly registered nurses are also consistent with those experienced by other health professionals and you may even feel as though you are an imposter like Marek in the scenario (Mandy and Tinley, 2004; Morley, 2009; Kearns, 2016).

The adjustment from education to full-time practice and the nurse's ability to integrate themselves in their new environment will hasten the transition and lessen the shock. From the moment nurses are registered, they are autonomous, accountable practitioners (NMC, 2015). It is clear then that those feelings of stress and fear felt during this time are often linked to high expectations of yourself and how you will meet your own and others' expectations. There is then a need for a newly registered nurse to form functional relationships with colleagues, to be integrated into the ward team and subsequently to develop into the role.

The following case study from an interview of a GP by Hugh Kearns demonstrates the impact of transition.

Case study

Entering general practice training as a junior registrar was a completely different story. With just you, the patient, and a supervising specialist GP watching your progress, you are completely exposed. And this, coupled with the fact that junior registrars are going to make mistakes, made for a very humbling experience. I couldn't count the number of times I reached the conclusion that being a doctor was just not for me. I regularly thought about my 'fall back' options, going back to research, perhaps teaching, or maybe stacking shelves at the supermarket.

Activity 7.1 Reflection

On a piece of paper write down how you are feeling now about your transition, reflecting on the case study above. Now go to your SWOT analysis formulated from Chapter 2 and reflect on what you have found.

As this activity is based upon your own reflection, there is no outline answer at the end of the chapter.

By getting you to reflect on the GP's story and your SWOT analysis above we wanted you to be able to distinguish whether you were a real imposter. We hope you have gathered that you are not, as a real imposter is a person who pretends to be someone else in order to deceive others, especially for fraudulent gain; whereas once you see your SWOT it will help you to realise how competent you are. What you may be sensing are imposter feelings; that is, feelings that you are a fraud, and when you explore the facts you are not. If you continue to feel like an imposter a lot of the time despite evidence to the contrary such as Marek in the scenario and this affects how you think and behave, you may have developed imposter syndrome. In this instance, you need to seek help. Table 7.1 lists imposter breaking strategies by Thinkwell that you may wish to consider.

You will note that reservations and worries can hold us back, so the best strategy when you are beginning to feel like an imposter is to act. For example, if we refer to Marek in

1	**Realise that imposter feelings are normal**
	Most people have imposter feelings from time to time. It's normal to question yourself, to ask how you're going. Then you need to look at the evidence.
2	**Know your imposter moments**
	There will be times when you are more likely to experience imposter feelings. If you know your imposter moments, then you can prepare yourself.
3	**Objective standards of success**
	Before you start on a project or task, write down what you would consider a success. This will stop you changing the goalposts later.
4	**Setting realistic standards**
	Set goals and standards that you can achieve. If you set outrageous standards, it makes failure more likely and you might avoid starting at all.
5	**Prepare for mistakes**
	Mistakes can stir up imposter feelings. Since mistakes are inevitable, it is a good idea to prepare yourself. Expect to feel annoyed but then decide what you will do.
6	**Mind your language**
	Stick to the facts. Was it just good luck or did you work hard? Did others do all the work or did you contribute too?
7	**Get external evidence**
	Rather than just relying on your opinions, seek out evidence, ask others, get facts.
8	**Do some behavioural experiments**
	Try things out to see whether your assumptions are true, for example when in practice ask for feedback on the care you give or clinical decisions you make.
9	**Create a fact file**
	Write down the facts in a fact file. Use this when an imposter moment strikes.
10	**Create a brag file**
	This will help you keep a record of your achievements and positive feedback.
11	**Remember that you are in charge**
	Even though they may be compelling, remember feelings are not facts.

Table 7.1 Imposter breaking strategies

the scenario, Marek should have understood that feeling like an imposter was normal. Using reflection to help, Marek could have identified that feeling anxious prior to each shift because of fear of not knowing how to respond to the demands of patients and members of the interprofessional team were 'imposter moments'. By using personal development planning with support from a preceptor, Marek could identify long- and short-term goals in relation to fear of not knowing how to respond to the demands of others and used objective feedback to measure success.

Setting realistic goals, with actions and resources that address who to ask and how to ask for feedback that reflects both personal progression and what to do when things go wrong, Marek could assess professional development and ability to cope. This would be from factual information, rather than a personal, one-sided emotional response. The benefits of a PDP also allows Marek to create a 'brag and fact' file that visibly demonstrates achievements during the period of preceptorship. Please refer back to Chapter 3 for further information.

The physical presence of a supporting individual (moving from mentorship to preceptorship/transition support)

Concept summary

What is a preceptorship/transitional support programme? How is it different to mentorship?

To support the transition from student nurse to newly registered nurse many healthcare settings have adopted a Staff Nurse Preceptorship Programme. The NMC (2006) defines preceptorship *as a period to guide and support all newly qualified practitioners to make the transition from student to develop their practice further.*

Preceptorship is not a new concept, the need for support was formally recognised in the UK in 1986 and professional bodies at this time recommended a period of learning after registration followed by a lifelong programme of continuing education. The drivers to implement supportive structures for newly registered nurses were based on two main features: to alleviate the transitional challenges of new practitioners to reduce the number of newly registered nurses leaving nursing as soon as they qualify, and a concern about the fitness to practice of newly registered practitioners.

Since 1986 there have been key documents that have ensured preceptorship has remained a recommendation for sound professional practice. The table below provides three key external drivers that promote the need for preceptorship. However, as all guidance on preceptorship is optional and not mandatory, some employers may offer a preceptorship programme, whereas others offer other forms of transition support.

In 2010 the Department of Health launched a 'preceptorship framework for newly registered nurses, midwifes and allied health professionals' to set clear standards for preceptorship.

Preceptorship is therefore a system put in place to support the transition phase for newly registered nurses as they continue their professional development, building confidence and further developing competence to practise and provide structure and direction. Preceptorship continues to feature as a priority as the Shape of Caring Review (Willis Commission, 2012) has recommended 1-year preceptorship with an employer following registration. Preceptorship is an integral part of enabling a newly registered nurse to practise safely unsupervised. As such it is a very important part of the development and transition route to independent practice; the programme may feature completion of mandatory workbooks, reflections and study days (to name some activities). Failure to advance at the two progression points within the first six to twelve months of a preceptorship programme could compromise a nurse's career or registration.

At the interim and end of the preceptorship period reviews should be held. The discussion at the reviews should not come as a surprise to the preceptee as feedback should be consistent throughout the programme with regular feedback on progress. If the preceptee has not provided sufficient evidence that they have met the required standards, the line manager as well as the preceptor will record which of the standards or performance criteria have not yet been achieved and provide detailed feedback to the preceptee. This will be recorded both in the preceptorship and appraisal documents. At this point it is the line manager who will decide locally whether human resources advice and support should be sought. At this time consideration will be given to either extend the preceptorship period or follow the trust/organisations competency policy; this may include contacting the Nursing and Midwifery Council under Fitness to Practice if the incidents or ill health issues are serious and compromise patient safety.

Organisation	Driver
Care Quality Commission	Competent
Staff – Standard 14	Registration requirements states we must take all reasonable steps to ensure that workers are appropriately supported to enable them to deliver care safely and to an appropriate standard
Department of Health	Developing the Healthcare Workforce; DoH preceptorship framework (for newly registered nurses, midwives and allied health professionals March 2010)
Nursing and Midwifery Council	Recommendation 21 of the NMC's 'Fitness to Practice'

Table 7.2 Key external drivers

When you are considering which staff nurse post to apply for or attending job interviews it is wise to discover whether your prospective employers have a preceptorship programme in place. Ask how long it lasts and what it will include, consider whether this programme will be of benefit to you, will it address your development needs. Cross-reference the programme against your SWOT analysis formulated in Chapter 2. For further information on applying for a staff nurse job see Chapter 8.

It is important that the programme you select is suitable for your needs as preceptorship programmes can be varied. Robinson and Griffiths (2008) and Chapman (2013) called for preceptorship programmes that fit the needs of the individual and should be a way to build confidence and further develop competence and not as a way to meet any shortfall in pre-registration education (DoH, 2010).

The need for a preceptorship/support programme is acknowledged in policy, though details of what is needed are sometimes unclear. Literature demonstrates a variance in length and content of both preceptorship and support programmes and authors have found difficulties in identifying individual learning needs of newly registered nurses (Evans, Boxer and Sanber, 2008; Darvill, 2013, Strauss *et al.*, 2015).

You may find that support programmes on offer vary in length, content and structure, it is a good idea to discuss the details of any support programme during your interview, that way you may find your 'right fit'. Some nurses may prefer a more structured programme such as their experience during nurse education, which focusses on attaining specific clinical competencies; however, some nurses may prefer the programme to focus on other important aspects of preceptorship such as peer support/networking and socialisation. A recommendation made by the National Nursing Research Unit (Robinson and Griffiths, 2008) concludes that any formal Structured Nurse Preceptorship programme should be speciality specific, and tailored toward the individual nurse's needs.

The support programme you choose should provide a supportive function, as if it became a task it could add more pressure to an already stressful time and serve to have the opposite effect to the supportive, developmental programme it set out to be. Some degree of formal outcomes such as developing your competencies may, however, be beneficial in developing the skills pertinent to your new role. Therefore, the programme you choose should be a balanced period of support and needs to be specific, individualised and not overly onerous. The Department of Health (DoH) is specific when it states that *the programme should be seen as a way to build confidence and further develop competence and not as a way to meet any shortfall in pre-registration education* (DoH, 2010, p10). It is now time for you to think: What do I want from my support programme? You may wish to read the systematic review that is included in the further reading section of this chapter.

Now that you have surveyed and reflected on your needs during your transition it is important to explore self-confidence. According to the literature, self-confidence could be your perception of your ability to interact with patients, families and colleagues

Activity 7.2   Reflection

Now that you have read more about preceptorship/transition support what do you think you would want/need to be included in your preceptorship/support?

Review your Personal Development Portfolio, Practice Assessment Document, or a Band 5 Job Description & Specification. Undertake a SWOT analysis (as demonstrated in Chapter 2) which will help you to identify actual/potential areas for development that should be included in your transition support programme.

While writing your list you may have used the word 'competent' and the word 'confidence'. What do you understand by the term confidence and the term competence? Write down your answer.

Consider how the preceptorship/transition support programme can develop your self-confidence and your clinical competence.

You will find an outline answer at the end of the chapter.

and safely carry out your new role in the clinical setting. Competence however, predicates the application of your knowledge and skills in responding appropriately to the dynamic patient-care environment (Roach, 2002). You could say that when you develop and safely demonstrate your competence you will then increase your confidence. The preceptor or support individual is charged with the role of guiding newly registered nurses and helping them to apply theory in practice; when you work with your preceptor/support person and demonstrate to them your competence, then this will help you to develop your confidence.

Supernumerary period

Supernumerary status means that you are additional to the clinical workforce and will spend time as such. A preceptorship/transition programme may allow a newly registered nurse to have time in the clinical area as a supernumerary member of staff. This will enable you to spend periods working with your preceptor/support person to learn from them and not as a member of staff with an allocated work load. This status would allow you attend study days where you will learn and develop alongside a group of your peers away from the clinical area, you may also be expected to complete specific outcomes and competencies that your employer has identified to help you to develop basic knowledge, skills and attitudes to perform your new role. This will enable you to build on the knowledge, skills and competences acquired as students in your chosen area of practice, laying a solid foundation for lifelong learning. The length of time your supernumerary status lasts can be anything from 15 days to a month. However, this is dependent on many variables such as appraisal of your current knowledge and skills and how quickly you adapt to the new clinical role.

Role of the preceptor/support person

A preceptor/support person has been defined as a registered practitioner who has been given formal responsibility to support a newly registered practitioner through preceptorship (DoH, 2010, p6).

As a student nurse, you would have worked closely with a mentor during each clinical placement. Working with a preceptor/support person should allow you to receive both support and education. There are however some small differences in the two roles. A mentor is required to undergo training and holds a qualification to perform the role. Currently there is no specific preparation for the role of preceptor/support person. If you are familiar with the differences this may help you to get the best from your preceptor.

Although your mentor would have been responsible for verifying your competence as a student the preceptor/support person will be there to help you consolidate your learning and support you through the transitional process to become an autonomous practitioner. Working alongside your preceptor/support person you will observe how they demonstrate their professional attributes, such as communication skills, problem solving, prioritising and decision making; you could look upon your preceptor/support person as a role model.

You may have noted that the ability to give constructive feedback is the first attribute a preceptor/support person should possess. It is therefore important to explore what feedback, the types of feedback, how to receive it and what to do with it.

Scenario: Marek and Gayle

If we look once again at how Marek and Gayle developed their preceptor/preceptee relationship we can appreciate that each preceptee will have individual development needs and will require varying levels of support to help consolidate their learning through the transitional process toward becoming an autonomous practitioner. By working alongside Gayle, Marek was able to observe how Gayle demonstrates professional attributes such as communication skills, problem solving, prioritising and decision making; you could look upon the preceptor/support person as a role model. Gayle also provided support by simply taking time to talk with Marek, answer questions and offer guidance and feedback, this resulted in Marek feeling confident in the new role to seek out further development opportunities independently.

Activity 7.3   Reflection

Imagine your ideal preceptor/support person. Perhaps you have someone in mind that supported you as a student nurse! What personal and professional attributes would/should they have and how and why would this benefit you?

You will find an outline answer at the end of the chapter.

Feedback – why is this important?

Let's go back to the initial scenario of Marek: in order for Marek to advance in knowledge and skill development Marek required constructive feedback from Gayle. As a student, Marek would be aware of the concept of assessment and feedback in relation to meeting the requirements in both theory and practice across the duration of their pre-registration nursing programme. Marek would then find it difficult if feedback was not forthcoming in the new role as a registered nurse.

A dictionary definition of feedback is information about reactions to a person's performance of a task, which is used as a basis for improvement. However, as a newly registered nurse, feedback is considered detailed information about the assessment between a trainee's observed performance and a standard; given with the goal to advance the trainee's performance (Van der Ridder *et al.*, 2008). In Marek's case feedback was important, in order to assess Marek's competence against the job roles and responsibilities of a registered nurse on a general medical ward.

Constructive feedback is the method of offering feedback about knowledge, skills and attitudes that are below the required level of competence and ability with the aim to improve it. It can involve informing the newly registered nurse of the standard required and/or providing them with suggestions about how to meet them.

Unconstructive feedback, however, is the process of providing feedback to a newly registered nurse deprived of any intention of improving their knowledge, skills or attitudes. This type of feedback is negative, often destructive, and should be avoided.

Constructive feedback should be:

- based on observed skills and behaviour;
- given on a regular basis;
- both verbal and written;
- full of probing questions about the newly registered nurse's own assessment of their knowledge, skills and values;
- related to current skill and knowledge level and desired goals;
- clear and focussed;

- positive and promote a change in performance and meeting of learning objectives/skills;
- given in sizeable chunks so any changes can be addressed in a systematic way, too much information and the newly registered nurse may feel overwhelmed;
- socialising the newly registered nurse to the profession;
- specific with information about desired improvements or corrective changes alongside a supporting rationale;
- based around further actions for the newly registered nurse to work towards as part of either an action plan or appraisal process. For example: being provided with opportunities to develop your knowledge, skills and experiences; being allocated workload based on previous experience and capability level; being given the autonomy to work independently to gain confidence through experience;
- encouraging reflective questioning in order to develop the newly registered nurse's critical thinking and decision-making skills that can help them to analyse current knowledge, skills, attitudes;
- given in private whenever possible;
- a two-way process so the newly registered nurse can share their views on the feedback they have just received (Duffy, 2013).

As you may have noticed, feedback is a complex process; therefore any information provided needs to be meaningful and clearly linked to competencies set out in the transition/preceptorship programme.

The Preceptorship Framework for Newly Registered Nurses, Midwives and Allied Health Professionals (DoH, 2010) suggests that all newly registered staff joining an organisation should have at least two development reviews within the first 12 months of employment. The purpose of these assessments is to establish the progress a preceptee is making towards criteria and competencies defined by the line manager and linked to indicators such as those in the KSF (DoH, 2004). This allows for the objective measurement and feedback of the preceptee's knowledge, skills, and attitudes by the preceptor; for example, using an assessment of a preceptee against KSF Core Dimension 1: Communication. In this instance the appraisal by the preceptor would be based upon the nature and extent of the communicating in the preceptee's everyday job. Exploring manner, tone and words used when communicating. Preceptors may use the acronym DOVE: documents, observations, verbal and electronic (NHS Scotland, 2010) to provide them with evidence to measure how the newly registered nurse has met the indicator or competence as found in Table 7.3.

While positive, negative and constructive feedback can enhance learning, unconstructive feedback may have a detrimental effect on both personal and professional development. Providing no feedback can result in a false level of security for the newly registered nurse. They may think they are doing well and have an enhanced sense of confidence and are not having any of their knowledge, skills and attitudes observed and reflected upon. This can subsequently affect patient care as unsupported newly registered nurses often hesitate to ask questions or seek advice as they feel they are not

Core dimension/ Clinical competence	Examples of how the dimension or competence will be met	Date met
KSF core dimension 1: Communication	*Documents:* forms and documents, for example, risk assessments, care plans, treatment records, completed order records, letters and thank you notes from patients, reflective accounts.	
	Observations: carrying out tasks, talking with colleagues, patients and others, reporting incidents.	
	Verbal: question and answer sessions on current policies and procedures, discussions on scenarios.	
	Electronic: e-learning achievements and presentations.	

Table 7.3 Examples of evidence used for a development review

coping or not able. This can end in errors and incidents where the quality of patient care is affected. Unconstructive feedback, however, usually lacks detail, offers no recommendations for how knowledge, skills and attitudes can be improved, and uses rude words or ones with negative connotations. It is often intended to offend and can include undeserved, personal attacks, leaving the newly registered nurse defensive.

Receiving feedback

It is important to consider the skills needed to receive feedback whether that be good or not so good. Listening carefully and being open to what is being said, making sure you have fully understood this before deciding on how you will respond. To ensure you have fully understood the feedback ask specific questions to avoid any misunderstanding and to clarify the points being made. Try to frame questions to get as much information as possible to ensure improvement in the future; e.g. when I did this I should have … is this correct? Not all feedback will be positive, therefore the newly registered nurse needs to be aware of the emotional effect that feedback may generate, particularly if this is not as positive as expected. There needs to be some self-awareness and self-control if feedback causes an emotional response, therefore some understanding of emotional intelligence is essential. For example, you can respond to feedback in four main ways:

Defensive: where you see the feedback as a personal attack aimed at your personal identity, and your emotions respond as though it was a threat to your existence. Being defensive means the feedback is often ignored, denied and creates anger and retaliation. By reacting this way, you will not learn anything and severely affect the preceptor–preceptee relationship.

Dispirited: where you take on board every piece of feedback without checking to see whether this is factually correct and supported. Responding to feedback in this way creates a strong emotional response, viewed as a personal attack and demoralising. This then leads to a refusal to learn or to change one's behaviour.

Dismissive: when feedback is not taken seriously, an assumption is made that the feedback given is wrong, or the person giving feedback is not to be trusted. It does not create an emotional response, but there is no engagement with the opportunity to learn from the feedback given.

Open: reacting to feedback in an open way allows you to reflect on your recollection of the behaviour or actions, check on the facts and take the criticism or praise on board.

Remember that your first response to feedback may change when you have had the opportunity to examine it in a more detached way later. By being open to feedback you can assess whether the facts are correct and make allowances for the skills of the person who delivered it. In the next activity we would like you to reflect on some feedback you have received as a student and how with time you may have changed your response to it.

Activity 7.4   Reflection

Think back to when you received constructive feedback in the past, for example from a lecturer on a piece of theoretical assessment you had submitted, or feedback from your mentors/personal tutor about your knowledge and skills. Which of the four main ways did you initially respond to receiving that feedback? Now that time has passed, review the facts and the skills of the person who delivered it. Has your response changed?

As this activity is based on individual experiences there is no outline answer at the end of the chapter.

The 'feedback sandwich'

Feedback is more likely to be accepted and acted upon if it is seen to be 'balanced' in that it is neither overly critical nor positive but provides a clear indication of the good and not so good. The 'sandwich' presents any negative aspects of feedback between two positives that offers a more balanced approach to the feedback process (Dohrenwend, 2002). For example; your written plans of care have improved and are more specific and focussed than when you started … your numeracy skills still need some work, specifically around intravenous fluid rates as you continue to have problems with this. I can really tell that you care about developing yourself as a nurse.

Networks and resources

In Chapter 4 you explored accessing support to maintain your personal health and wellbeing from the family and friends activities feature as a support mechanism to help ensure you kept physically and mentally well. In the workplace, however, there are other networks and resources that as a newly registered nurse you can call upon to support you during your transition.

Other members of the nursing team (registered and support workers) in the workplace can be a valuable resource to assist in easing your transition. Develop what is called your 'social capital' (Melling, 2011) by taking opportunities to build good social relationships. Watch other staff members closely, pay attention to how they work and complete tasks. Some will be excellent role models of how you should conduct yourself while at work and the skills required to provide a quality service. Ask for their advice and help when you are unsure and remember to thank them when they have helped, to show your appreciation.

Other members of the interprofessional team are another helpful resource. Often when newly registered nurses qualify, members of other professions are new registrants also. Take time to get to know who the members of the interprofessional team are, seek their help when you know your limitations, ask them to show you or teach you aspects of their role that may be of benefit to your own knowledge, skills and attitudes. Again, always remember to thank others for their help and support.

Clinical nurse educators can assist your transition with helping to provide practical and skills-oriented training under the supervision of a skilled practitioner.

Study days are encouraged and often a requirement as part of your transitional period. This is for you to develop the skills and knowledge necessary to competently carry out your role, demonstrate that you remain fit to practice and have the necessary skills to provide patients with the highest level of care. Study days, conferences and seminars serve to inform your professional knowledge, by sharing research and best practice – crucial to learning and building up an evidence base from which to draw upon. During your attendance at study days you will also meet other newly registered nurses and staff who can increase your circle of support networks.

Peer support groups are often organised as part of preceptorship/transition support programmes. Support from these groups includes emotional support, new insights and rewards. Peer groups also give encouragement and optimism when you become stressed by the emotional labour of nursing and some of the clinical decisions you have made.

Autonomous decisions about clinical judgements, choices and actions

According to the Royal College of Nursing (2014, p3):

Nursing is the use of clinical judgement in the provision of care to enable people to improve, maintain, or recover health, to cope with health problems, and to achieve the best possible quality of life, whatever their disease or disability, until death.

To carry this out a nurse must develop and demonstrate autonomy and control over their nursing practice. This in turn has been linked with increased job satisfaction and improved patient outcomes. As a newly registered nurse, a programme of support is needed so that you may develop these skills required to become an autonomous practitioner and make clinical judgements about patient care safely and with support from your preceptor and other registered nurses within the clinical area.

Autonomy and accountability are two major issues that newly registered nurses worry about. However, in order to make effective clinical decisions, which in nursing occur several times a day, newly registered nurses should use information they have gathered using tools of assessment, theoretical knowledge, general awareness and experience to inform the process. Good clinical decision making requires an amalgamation of skills that include: pattern recognition from learning experiences, critical thinking, communication skills using active listening, evidence based practices, team work, sharing and discussion of your decisions with others and reflection.

Concept summary

According to Weston (2010) autonomy represents the ability to act according to one's knowledge and judgement, delivering care within one's scope of practice as outlined in current professional, regulatory, and organisational rules. The Nursing and Midwifery Council (2010), as part of the standards for pre-registration education, state that a competency required prior to entry on the professional register is that nurses *must practise autonomously and be responsible and accountable for safe, compassionate, person-centred, evidence-based nursing that respects and maintains dignity and human rights.*

Strategies that will help you to become autonomous/independent will include: your preceptor describing expected behaviours and providing opportunity to practise behaviours; senior staff recognising and rewarding your positive behaviours; you role modelling behaviours of autonomy and independence observed; and your support person/preceptor providing constructive feedback when you do not demonstrate positive behaviours.

NHS Scotland (2010) recognised four issues that can have an impact on clinical decision making; these include: knowing the evidence in order to be able to deal with the current patient or situation; knowing yourself and how your and others' attitudes, values, beliefs and behaviour can impact the care delivered; knowing the patient and their experience, knowledge and current situation in regard to their illness; knowing the environment in order for you to take a considered approach to the decision-making process which may mean bearing in mind team dynamics, ward culture and personalities. For example, you have been asked to carry out a dressing change on a patient with a surgical wound. Using the four issues approach, your ability to care for the patient and their wound would depend upon:

- your knowledge of anatomy and physiology of the skin and the process of wound healing;
- your knowledge and skills of completing wound assessments, wound cleansing techniques and choosing the right dressing;
- your reaction to the wound appearance, odour and/or leakage;
- where you will undertake the dressing change on the ward and do you need assistance;
- who can help and what time you will change the dressing.

A prescriptive method that nurses use to help with clinical decision making is a four-stage process of assessment, planning, implementation and evaluation (Yura and Walsh, 1973). To complete these stages effectively you must consider all assessments and their results using look, listen and feel, then make judgements on the data collected, what is happening, decide what to do, include colleagues in your discussions and evaluate the outcome of the decision. It is important during your preceptorship that you consider activities that will help you to achieve these skills. If you wish to read more about the topic of clinical decision making there are other books in the transforming nursing practice series addressing this topic in some depth such as Standing (2017). A useful way to start to address your skills in clinical decision making is to write a list.

Activity 7.5 Decision making

Considering your new job as a newly registered nurse what activities could you ask to be involved in to develop your autonomy and enhance your decision-making skills.

You will find an outline answer at the end of the chapter.

Now you have reflected on the activities you could ask to be involved in to develop autonomy and enhance your decision making, the next section explores what support you could ask for once your preceptorship/transition support ends.

Clinical supervision

Once the period of preceptorship/transition support has ended, you may feel as though there is no further support for your development. However, many organisations offer clinical supervision. This is defined by the Royal College of Nursing (2002, p1) as:

an activity that brings skilled supervisors and practitioners together in order to reflect upon their practice. It is a time for you, as a nurse or midwife, to think about your knowledge and skills and how they may be developed to improve care.

Chapter summary

By reading this chapter we hope that you will be able to comprehend what transition support now means. By completing the reading and activities you should now be able to recognise what to expect in relation to transition support when you commence employment in your new role as a registered nurse. You should also now be able to identify the need for supernumerary status at the start of your job and describe the different types of feedback and recognise the impact this has on job performance. Finally, identifying other networks and resources that can assist with transition support and recognising when you are ready to start to make autonomous decisions about clinical judgements, choices and actions.

Activities: brief outline answers

Activity 7.2 Reflection (page 143)

Competence: the delivery of safe care to a required standard.

Confidence: confidence is an internal feeling of self-assurance and comfort. Confidence as a nurse comes from experience and exposure to as many different patient scenarios and clinical situations as possible.

Activity 7.3 Reflection (page 145)

Here is a list of attributes of a preceptor developed by the Department of Health. Which of these attributes did you consider?

- the ability to give constructive feedback;
- setting goals and assessing competency;
- facilitating problem solving;
- active listening skills;

- understanding, demonstrating and evidencing reflective-practice ability in the working environment;
- demonstrating good time management and leadership skills;
- prioritising care;
- demonstrating appropriate clinical decision making and evidence-based practice;
- recognising their own limitations and those of others;
- knowing what resources are available and how to refer to a preceptee appropriately, if the preceptee needs additional support;
- being an effective role model and demonstrating professional values, attitude and behaviours;
- demonstrating a clear understanding of the regulatory impact of the care that they deliver and the ability to pass on this knowledge.

Activity 7.5 Decision making (page 151)

Activities that can enable your development of autonomy and clinical decision making include: observing and then participating in ward rounds; observing senior nurses and role models; coaching from your preceptor; attending and participating in staff meetings, case conferences, and best interest's meetings etc. Then, as you become integrated into the ward team, being put forward for modules of study, study days, becoming a link nurse etc.

Further reading

Burns, D (2015) *Foundations of Adult Nursing*. Los Angeles, CA: Sage.

This essential book covers the issues, themes and principles that nurses practising today should be familiar with. Often aimed at student nurses this book also provides the registered nurse with an easily accessible reference to the issues key to your career. Similar books are also available for other fields of nursing.

Richards, A and Edwards, S (2013) *A Nurse's Survival Guide to the Ward* (3rd edn). Edinburgh, UK: Elsevier.

This is a useful guide to keep close at hand. It is an essential reference for nurses, not only on the ward but also in every field of practice where patient care is given.

Whitehead, B, Owen, P, Holmes, D, Beddingham, E, Simmons, M, Henshaw, L, Barton, M and Walker, C (2013) Supporting newly qualified nurses in the UK: A systematic literature review. *Nurse Education Today*, 33(4): 370–7.

This is a systematic review of the literature that enables you to know what a good preceptorship programme should look like.

Useful websites

Thinkwell – a website produced by researchers and practitioners in cognitive behavioural therapy who use the latest psychological and educational research to assist high achievers to achieve maximum productivity.

www.ithinkwell.com.au/index.php

Chapter 8

Preparing for, developing and maintaining your nursing career

Andy Kay, Leyonie Higgins and Angela Darvill

NMC Standards for Pre-registration Nursing Education

As this chapter is concerned with providing evidence of competence, its underlying principles relate to all four domains of the competencies:

Domain 1: Professional values

Generic standard for competence: All nurses must act first and foremost to care for and safeguard the public. They must practise autonomously and be responsible and accountable for safe, compassionate, person-centred, evidence-based nursing that respects and maintains dignity and human rights. They must show professionalism and integrity and work within recognised professional, ethical and legal frameworks. They must work in partnership with other health and social care professionals and agencies, service users, their carers and families in all settings, including the community, ensuring that decisions about care are shared.

Domain 2: Communication and interpersonal skills

Generic standard for competence: All nurses must use excellent communication and interpersonal skills. Their communications must always be safe, effective, compassionate and respectful. They must communicate effectively using a wide range of strategies and interventions including the effective use of communication technologies. Where people have a disability, nurses must be able to work with service users and others to obtain the information needed to make reasonable adjustments that promote optimum health and enable equal access to services.

Domain 3: Nursing practice and decision making

Generic standard for competence: All nurses must practise autonomously, compassionately, skilfully and safely, and must maintain dignity and promote health and wellbeing. They must assess and meet the full range of essential physical and mental health needs of people of all ages who come into their care. Where necessary they must be able to provide safe and effective immediate care to all people prior to accessing or referring to specialist services, irrespective of their field of practice. All nurses must also meet more complex and coexisting needs for people in their own nursing field of practice, in any setting including hospital, community and at home. All practice should be informed by the best available evidence and comply with local and national guidelines. Decision making must be shared with service users, carers and families and informed by critical analysis of a full range of possible interventions, including the use of up-to-date technology. All nurses must also understand how behaviour, culture, socio-economic and other factors, in the care environment and its location, can affect health, illness, health outcomes and public health priorities and take this into account in planning and delivering care.

Domain 4: Leadership, management and team working

Generic standard for competence: All nurses must be professionally accountable and use clinical governance processes to maintain and improve nursing practice and standards of healthcare. They must be able to respond autonomously and confidently to planned and uncertain situations, managing themselves and others effectively. They must create and maximise opportunities to improve services. They must also demonstrate the potential to develop further management and leadership skills during their period of preceptorship and beyond.

This chapter will address all five ESCs:

1. Care, compassion and communication (1–8)
2. Organisational aspects of care (9–20)
3. Infection prevention and control (21–26)
4. Nutrition and fluid management (27–32)
5. Medicines management (33–42)

Chapter aims

After reading this chapter and undertaking the activities, you will be able to:

- understand the recruitment process from the employers' perspective;
- analyse job descriptions and person specifications;
- complete an online application form and write a supporting statement;
- complete a CV if required;
- prepare for and take part in the interview or assessment day process;
- reflect on the interview process;
- access relevant online resources to start your nursing career.

Introduction

The purpose of this chapter is to help you secure your first nursing post. The chapter begins by enabling you to develop an understanding of the recruitment process and consider the evidence you will provide to meet your employers' expectations regarding your knowledge, skills and values to secure your first post. The chapter will begin by introducing a scenario based on a final year student considering applying for a post as a newly registered nurse. You will be able to review current job descriptions and person specifications and consider collating your evidence to enable you to write your application form. Specific requirements when applying for a job will be examined, including health, learning needs, declaration of convictions and fitness to practise. Guidance will be provided on preparing for interview and finally suggestions for continuing professional development will be discussed.

This chapter will introduce you to the job recruitment process and assist you in developing your application and personal specification. The chapter provides you with examples of job descriptions and enables you to consider collating evidence that can help you apply for your dream job. The chapter will also help you to understand how to declare your specific health and learning needs to your employer and consider how to declare any previous criminal or fitness to practice convictions. You will be able to consider your supporting statement that matches the job description and person specification. Then move on to preparing for the interview and taking part in the interview process. You can research possible interview questions and consider preparing and planning your responses. Finally, the chapter will enable you to consider planning and developing your learning and development needs for your continuing career.

Consider the following scenario:

Scenario: Nusrat

Nusrat is a final Year nursing student, who began the third year three months ago. At the beginning of Year 3 students were told to start applying for jobs sooner rather than later. Nusrat has thought about where to apply for jobs but does not know how to go about doing this yet. Nusrat has spoken to peers and some of them have applied for jobs already but have not been successful. The thought of applying is stressful, making Nusrat anxious. Nusrat knows the process of applying is lengthy and does not really know what to expect from the interviews. So far no one at the university has gone through the process of applying for jobs or told them how to make a start. Students are unclear whether this process is something they are going to get support with or they have to undertake on their own. If there are no jobs in the area, Nusrat is considering accepting whatever is available until an ideal job becomes available.

This chapter has started with the above scenario to help set the context of student nurses considering applying for their first post.

Understanding the recruitment process and making great applications

It is important to look at the recruitment process through the eyes of the employer. Employers are looking to recruit the right members of staff to care for patients and that they are safe, competent practitioners, fit for purpose and fit for practise. They also want nurses that can demonstrate care, compassion, dignity and respect. At the end of the day, they are looking for the best person to care for patients and will have three main questions in their mind about you.

1. Can you do the job they are recruiting for and will you be competent?
2. Will you fit into the team?
3. Do you share and demonstrate the values of the trust and the profession?

You can view the recruitment process as a funnel with the aim of continuously reducing the number of candidates until there is just one, or a small number of applicants who would be considered appointable. Given the number of potential applicants to a post, the employer will be keen to make the number manageable. It is important to note here that some vacancies can close early if enough applications have been received. Figure 8.1 demonstrates the recruitment process.

Let's think back to Nusrat and that confusion around the process of applying for jobs. Nusrat has a good idea about looking at NHS Jobs on www.jobs.nhs.uk and is using the site to explore the range of jobs available locally. This is a great start and you can get a good idea of which Trusts are recruiting and to what posts. The thing that is confusing is the amount of information that is provided. This includes job descriptions, person specifications and all the additional documentation that is often provided by the employer in order to give more information to the candidate. You will need to consider what is important in all of this and how to approach completing your application – ask yourself 'What information do I need to provide'? 'How can I make sure my applications are the best they can be'?

The key documents to focus on are the *job description* and the *person specification*. These documents are linked but serve different functions:

- The job description provides you with information about the job, i.e. the range of duties and responsibilities that go with the post. In other words, it tells you about the job you will be doing.

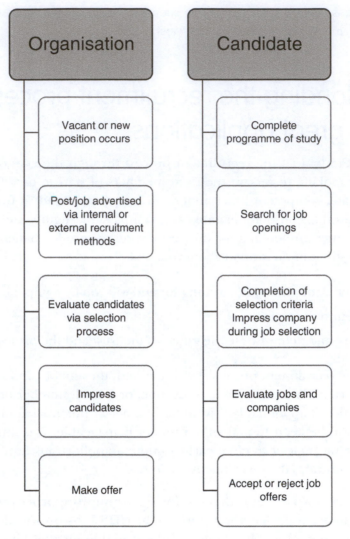

Figure 8.1   The recruitment process

- The person specification sets out the mix of skills, knowledge, experience and personal attributes that are required to carry out the duties and responsibilities outlined in the job description. It describes what you should have that will enable you to do the job.

For the employer it forms the basis of their scoring sheet, enabling objective judgements to be made on the quality of evidence provided by you to show how you meet the criteria for the post.

The following activity will enable you to explore the information on a current job description and begin to consider how you will use the job description to formulate your application.

Activity 8.1 Critical thinking

The job description

Access a job description from the NHS Jobs site and begin to note the evidence you can present that will demonstrate that you have the knowledge, skills, values and experience that the recruiter is looking for.

There is an outline answer to this activity at the end of the chapter.

Hopefully you find this a useful exercise and continue to collate evidence for all the statements on the job description. This evidence can form the basis for your application.

The person specification

For you, it is the person specification that is the key document within the recruitment process. It tells you exactly what you should be focusing on within your supporting statement. Each element of the person specification will be designated as 'essential' or 'desirable' and in turn there will be a key that will tell you how the element will be assessed. Commonly the methods used will be indicated as follows:

AF = Application Form

I = Interview

T = Test

R = References

Although every employer in the NHS and the vast majority of private providers will use job descriptions and person specifications, it is important to recognise that these are not standard across employers. The job being advertised may largely be the same in two different trusts but the content and appearance of the person specification can be radically different.

Figure 8.2 shows an example of a typical person specification:

You need to understand the importance of meeting the essential criteria and demonstrating an ability to work towards the desirable. However, you might not always meet everything on the person specification, but this shouldn't stop you from applying.

Every aspect of the person specification will be assessed at some point during the recruitment process. To be invited to interview or an assessment day you will need to provide the evidence of how you meet the criteria listed in the person specification. You will do this in different ways. Activity 8.2 will help you to begin completing your person specification.

REQUIREMENTS	CRITERIA	ESSENTIAL/ DESIRABLE	HOW ASSESSED?
1 Education/ Qualifications/ Training	• NMC Registered Nurse	E	AF
	• Assessing and Mentoring qualification	D	AF
	• Evidence of ongoing professional development linked to demonstrable competencies	D	AF
2 Skills/Abilities	• Ability to plan and prioritise care for patients	E	I
	• Articulates compassion when caring	E	I
	• Excellent verbal and written communication skills	E	AF/I
	• Good time management and teaching skills	E	I
	• Ability to work well both in a team and on own initiative	E	I
3 Experience	• Demonstrable experience as a student nurse in an acute setting	E	AF/I
	• Experience of having worked with acute/chronically ill patients	E	AF/I
	• Experience of supervising and assessing students	D	AF/I
	• Previous experience in the relevant specialty	D	AF/I
4 Knowledge	• Understanding of professional and current issues in nursing	E	I
	• Understanding of the importance of research and evidence based practice	E	I
	• Understanding of nursing practice and innovation	E	I
	• Knowledge of the clinical speciality	D	I
	• Awareness of cultural needs	E	I
	• Basic knowledge of computer skills	E	AF
5 Other requirements	• Good interpersonal skills	E	AF/I
	• A professional approach to work	E	AF/I
	• Willing to support others	E	AF/I
	• Demonstrates ability to use initiative	E	AF/I
	• Ability to work internal rotation to night duty (as appropriate)	E	AF/I
	Accountability – Takes responsibility for own actions and promotes good team working	E	AF/I
	Openness – Shares information and good practice appropriately	E	AF/I
	Mutual respect – Treats others with courtesy and respect at all times	E	AF/I
	Numerate – Able to demonstrate numeracy skills	E	T

Figure 8.2 Example of person specification

Activity 8.2   Decision making

Look at the person specification in Figure 8.2 and use the template in Table 8.1 below to organise your evidence:
Using the skills and abilities section of the person specification identify the evidence that you would provide for the criteria.

You could review your self-assessments that you have undertaken from Chapter 2 and use the outcomes of this to identify your Knowledge, Skills and Values.

Skills/Abilities	Evidence/Examples
Ability to plan and prioritise care for patients	
Good time management and teaching skills	
Ability to work well both in a team and on own initiative	

Table 8.1   The recruitment process

An outline answer for this activity is provided at the end of the chapter.

You will see from the outline answer that it is important to provide evidence for these criteria and not opinion statements. For example, statements that begin with 'I feel' or, 'I believe'.

Now continue this activity and note potential examples that you can use to illustrate how you meet each criterion.

Once the person specification and job description have been reviewed you can then begin to consider the application form.

The application form

The NHS online application form and others that you will complete will provide you with space to list your educational qualifications, your employment history, training courses attended among other things, but the key section of your application will be the supporting information. The key word to remember here is 'evidence'.

Declaring previous convictions

You will need to declare these on the job application form, as any offer made will be subject to satisfactory enhanced Disclosure and Barring Service (DBS) clearance.

Failure to disclose any convictions, cautions, reprimands, or warnings and any current criminal investigations taking place may put any offer of a job and your NMC registration at risk. You may wish to provide further information, it is always best to be open and honest.

This information will allow the interview panel to consider:

- nature and gravity of the offence(s);
- age at the time of the offence(s);
- length of time since the offence(s);
- number of offences;
- any pattern of offences;
- the severity of the sentence;
- relevance of offence(s) to profession;
- your response to offence(s) and rehabilitation;
- public trust.

Declaration of any Fitness to Practise (FtP) hearing during your programme of study

If the application form states: *Have you EVER been subject to a fitness to practise procedure* regardless of the outcome and consequences you need to be open and honest and act with integrity at all times. Consider including a statement about the circumstances of your FtP, the outcome and what you have done to reflect to ensure that you abide by the NMC code. Prospective employers will appreciate your honesty. You should also contact your Higher Education Institution (HEI) to enquire about what information regarding your FtP might be included in your academic reference.

Declaring specific health or learning needs

During the recruitment process, employers should ask whether you require any reasonable adjustments; this may be on the job advert or on the application form. The employer should not think that your requirement for reasonable adjustments means that you have a disability. Health-related questions are not allowed during interviews unless they are crucial to the role and what you are required to do. Employers should not discuss any adjustments you need to perform the role (these should only be discussed after a job offer is made) but can ask how you might undertake an essential part of the role with adjustments in place before they make an offer.

The Equality Act (2010) prevents discrimination because of disability, it covers conditions such as hearing and visual impairments, Specific Learning Difficulties (SpLD) and mental health difficulties; long-term health conditions such as diabetes, human immunodeficiency virus (HIV), multiple sclerosis (MS) epilepsy and cancer. The Equality Act places a duty on public authorities to promote equal opportunity and eliminate discrimination. Disclosure of a disability is a matter of personal choice; however, it is important that you consider your valid reasons for and against disclosure, but consider whether your employer is not aware of your disability – then the appropriate reasonable adjustments cannot be made. You may consider disclosing on your application:

- the nature of your disability;
- what reasonable adjustments have been put in place on your current programme of study;
- what personal strategies you use to enable you to manage your disability.

You may be reluctant to disclose your disability due to concerns about discrimination, but you should be reassured that the Equality Act (2010) makes provision for reasonable adjustments for you in the workplace. There are many advantages to disclosure:

- Taking responsibility for disclosure and managing your condition demonstrates professionalism.
- Demonstrating your skills such as the resourcefulness that having an impairment can bring is a good way of standing out from other candidates.
- You will be able to discuss with your employers the impact of your disability and the strategies you have developed to ensure that you are a competent practitioner.
- The employer will be able to ensure appropriate support is in place.
- Reasonable adjustments can be made that will allow you to reach your full potential as a newly registered nurse.
- Disclosure will allow you to focus on your preceptorship period.
- Disclosure will enable your employer to consider patients' and your health and safety needs.

If you choose not to disclose you need to consider that:

- your employer will not be able to ensure that you have the appropriate support in place to support your health or learning needs;
- it can become difficult to challenge discrimination or claim non-provision of support later on if you have chosen not to disclose.

Your supporting statement

It is at this point that many potentially good applicants become unstuck by submitting poorly structured supporting statements with generic content that expresses opinions rather than fact. Remember that the employer will be looking for you to provide specific evidence of how you meet the selection criteria. This means using the examples from Activity 8.2 that show how you have met the person specification. You will have identified examples of where you have demonstrated the application of your skills, knowledge and values and have proven that you have the requisite experience.

An important point to make here is that within the NHS application system you have a limit of 1,500 words for your supporting statement. This means that your statement needs to be focused, concisely written and devoid of waffle.

A suggested structure for your supporting statement is as follows:

1. Begin by writing an introductory paragraph outlining your reasons for applying for the post. You might also include some information that shows you have researched the Trust/clinical area, particularly the Trust values and the job role. You could also briefly cover how you see this post fitting in to a longer-term career plan. Ensure that you focus on the job here and not the fact that you have recently qualified and this job would be great because it's near where you live.

2. Using the headings provided in the person specification, follow the order of points as listed in the person specification. Depending on the number of points contained within the person specification (and these can vary widely in number), address each point providing specific evidence for each using the approach outline below. If the person specification contains a large number of criteria, then you will be needing to restrict your headings to the main sections and provide evidence that covers a number of points simultaneously. Be sure to follow the order of criteria as listed in the person specification.

3. Conclude with a short paragraph, restating your interest in the post and the Trust.

That's your structure but remember the employer will be looking for specifics. Once you have your evidence, you are ready to provide some short, focused statements that supply the information that the recruiter is looking for and it is here where the STAR or CAR approach can be useful.

STAR stands for:

S – Situation (when and where did this happen?)

T – Task (what did you have to do?)

A – Action (how did you do it?)

R – Result (what was the outcome?)

or if you prefer, CAR:

C – Context

A – Action

R – Result

CAR is a little bit simpler and just wraps up the situation and task into one part of your short statement.

Here is an example to demonstrate how the STAR/CAR approach can work for you:

Using CAR: Skills/abilities:

Ability to plan and prioritise care for patients.

C – The theoretical assessment in Year 2 semester 3 was about planning care for a patient newly diagnosed with diabetes. Within the assessment I was required to discuss assessment, implementation and evaluation of the patients care needs, ensuring care was patient centred.

A – I was able to put this learning into practice during the placement for that semester while …

R – I achieved a mark of 65% for the assessment, feedback stated …, the NMC competencies for that placement were achieved and my mentor commented …

Completing a CV

As a recent nursing graduate, you may need a CV. This won't usually be required as part of an application through NHS Jobs, but a CV can be asked for by agencies. Here is a template you might wish to use when putting together a nursing focused CV:

Use this template to start working on your CV:

Nusrat Student

10, Getwell Street, Anytown AN5 4TW

Tel: 0123 456 7890

Mob: 012345 123456

Email: n.student@edu.anytown.ac.uk

Career objective:

A concise statement of who you are, what you can offer and where you want to be, e.g.

'A highly motivated and enthusiastic xxxxxxxxx with high standards of holistic care seeking a challenging first post where I can use my maturity, skills and experience to make a valuable contribution to xxxxxxxxxxxxxxx'

Professional qualifications:

Provide some information about your nursing degree, i.e. name of institution, dates and expected degree result if known. Splitting your qualifications from your other qualifications provides an immediate focus on nursing.

Professional skills and experience:

This is the place to provide some information on the range of clinical placements undertaken. You can be selective here if you wish depending on the role applied for; for example, you might want to highlight specific experience in neonatal intensive care or within A&E etc. Alternatively, you might choose to provide an overview of the range of settings that you have worked in and provide a summary of the key skills, knowledge and professional behaviours demonstrated, e.g.:

- Worked effectively within a multi-disciplinary team: developed my professional skills and ability to work independently while managing a small caseload.
- Highly developed interpersonal skills gained through working alongside fellow professionals to practise family-centred care.
- Demonstrated care, compassion and empathy while supporting families through times of considerable stress.
- Wrote effective reports and documented interventions promptly and accurately.

Additional qualifications:

This is the section where any other educational qualifications can be listed, e.g. GCSEs, A-Level, other degree etc. Don't provide too much detail here, i.e. don't list all your GCSEs, it will be enough to write, '8 GCSEs grades A – C incl. Maths and English'.

Employment:

This section can be used to document any other work experience you may have. If not directly relevant to a healthcare setting, focus on transferable skills developed, e.g. communication, time management, planning and organisation, teamwork etc. and highlight any achievements that you consider to be important. You don't need to provide as much detail here. If you have been employed as a healthcare assistant during your studies, you could include that here.

Voluntary work:

This can also be a key section of your CV, particularly if you have range of voluntary experience that would be relevant to the role being sought. Your volunteer work can be viewed in the same way you would employment, i.e. an opportunity to highlight key skills and behaviours looked for by employers. Depending on the nature of your voluntary experience, this may well be a section that ranks above the employment section; if so, place the information within this section at an earlier point within your CV.

Additional information:

Include anything else that might be of interest here, e.g. training courses attended, driving licence, first aid certificates, language abilities, IT skills.

References:

Two referees are usually standard for a CV. For students these would normally comprise your tutor and a referee from a clinical setting. This should perhaps be someone of Band 6 or the ward manager. Alternatively, if you are limited in terms of space on your CV, you could simply write, 'References available on request'.

NB: It is important to recognise that your CV is a very flexible document. You may use all, or only some of the headings presented here. Use a format and structure that works best for you. Figure 8.3 will act as a guide when you come to complete the application form.

For Office Use Only
Online Reference Number:

NHS STANDARD APPLICATION FORM

(Please ensure that you read and follow instructions)

Please fill in the application form below using black ink. If typing do not use only capital letters and please remember to check it carefully, as once the form has been submitted it cannot be changed. Please note that questions marked with an asterisk * are mandatory and therefore must be answered.

APPLICATION FOR EMPLOYMENT WITH

APPLICATION FOR EMPLOYMENT Details entered in this part of the form will be held in the HR department of the recruiting organisation. Access to this information will be withheld from the shortlisting panel. Please do not type using only capital letters, as this could lead to your application being automatically rejected. Please use the appropriate mixture of capital and lowercase letters in standard written text.

Job Reference Number	It is important that you complete this so that Human Resources (HR) can ensure your application form gets to the right people
Job Title	E.g. Newly registered Band 5 staff nurse
Department	Full name of department if known (some posts may be rotational or for a job pool)

Personal Details

*Surname/Family Name	Given surname or married surname as documented on birth or marriage certificate
*First Names	First and middle names, as documented on birth/marriage certificate, passport or driving licence
Name in which you are registered with a professional body (if applicable)	
Title	E.g. Mr/Ms/Miss/Mrs/Dr
UK National Insurance No	This will prove that you are eligible to work in the UK
Address	Full address, please ensure that the ID information you bring matches the address you give here
*Postcode/ Zip code	
* Country	
Home Telephone	It is important that the interviews have correct current contact details in case they need to contact you urgently e.g. change of location or time
Mobile Telephone	As above
Work Telephone	

(Continued)

Figure 8.3 (Continued)

May we contact you at work?	☐　　Yes　　　☐　　　No
Email Address	Professional personal email address, or if you use your university email account make sure you check it regularly!

*Are you a United Kingdom (UK), European Community (EC) or European Economic Area (EEA) National?	
☐　　Yes　　☐　　No　　Employers need to know that you can legally work in the UK	

Please select the category that relates to your current immigration status. This status will be subject to checking before interview.

☐　HSMP/Tier 1	
☐　Indefinite Leave to remain/enter	☐　Post Graduate Doctors and Dentists
☐　Work Permit/Tier 2	☐　Tier 5 Temporary Workers
☐　Dependant/Spouse visa	☐　Working Holiday Visa/Tier 5 Youth Mobility
☐　Clinical attachment visa	☐　Refugee
☐　Student	
☐　Visitor	☐　Other, please specify below

Please supply details of any visa currently held, including number, start/expiry dates and details of any restrictions.

Visa No:

Start Date: (DD/MM/YY)

Expiry Date: (DD/MM/YY)

Details of Restriction:

This is only relevant if you have a visa that allows work in the UK

Does your visa have a condition restricting employment or occupation in the UK?

☐　　Yes　　☐　　No

Are you a Department of Work & Pensions New Deal Candidate?	☐　Yes　☐　No
Are you an NHS professional returning to practice?	☐　Yes　☐　No
Do you currently work in the NHS?	☐　Yes　☐　No

If you have a disability, do you require any reasonable adjustments to be made during the recruitment process, including interview?

☐　　Yes　　☐　　No see the information on pg... regarding the benefits of disclosure

If yes, please supply details below:

If you have a disability, do you wish to be considered under the Guaranteed Interview Scheme if you meet the minimum criteria as specified in the Person Specification?

☐　Yes　　☐　No

MONITORING INFORMATION Every year public organisations are required to publish data in relation to The Equality Act (2010) Pages 3–5 will give you an idea of the information that is collected. NB: As stated below, this information will not be seen by the selection panel.

This section of the application form will be detached from your application form. The information collected will only be used for monitoring purposes in an anonymised format and will help the organisation analyse the profile and make up of applicants and appointees to jobs in support of their equal opportunities policies.

NHS organisations recognise and actively promote the benefits of a diverse workforce and are committed to treating all employees with dignity and respect regardless of age, disability, gender reassignment, marriage and civil partnership, pregnancy and maternity, race, religion or belief, sex and sexual orientation. We therefore welcome applications from all sections of the community.

* Date of Birth	This will not be seen by the selection panel
* Gender	☐ Male
	☐ Female
	☐ I do not wish to disclose this

Equality Act 2010

* I would describe my ethnic origin as:		
Asian or Asian British	**Mixed**	**Other Ethnic Group**
☐ Bangladeshi	☐ White & Asian	☐ Chinese
☐ Indian	☐ White & Black African	☐ Any other ethnic group
☐ Pakistani	☐ White & Black Caribbean	☐ I do not wish to disclose this
☐ Any other Asian background	☐ Any other mixed background	
Black or Black British	**White**	
☐ African	☐ British	
☐ Caribbean	☐ Irish	
☐ Any other Black background	☐ Any other White background	

Equality Act 2010

* Please select the option which best describes your sexual orientation	
☐ Lesbian	
☐ Gay	☐ Heterosexual
☐ Bisexual	☐ I do not wish to disclose this

* Please indicate your religion or belief		
☐ Atheism	☐ Jainism	☐ Hinduism
☐ Buddhism	☐ Sikhism	☐ Other
☐ Christianity	☐ Judaism	☐ I do not wish to disclose this
☐ Islam		

(Continued)

Figure 8.3 (Continued)

Equality Act 2010

The Equality Act 2010 protects disabled people – including those with long term health conditions, learning disabilities and so called 'hidden' disabilities such as dyslexia. If you tell us that you have a disability we can make reasonable adjustments to ensure that any selection processes – including the interview – are fair and equitable.

* Do you consider yourself to have a disability?	☐ Yes
	☐ No
	☐ I do not wish to disclose this information
Please state the type of impairment which applies to you. People may experience more than one type of impairment, in which case you may indicate more than one. If none of the categories apply, please mark 'other'.	

☐ Physical impairment	☐ Learning disability/difficulty
☐ Sensory impairment	☐ Long-standing illness
☐ Mental health problem	☐ Other

Rehabilitation of Offenders Act 1974

The Rehabilitation of Offenders Act helps rehabilitated ex-offenders back into work by allowing them not to declare criminal convictions after the rehabilitation period set by the Court has elapsed and the convictions become 'spent'. During the rehabilitation period, convictions are referred to as 'unspent' convictions and must be declared to employers.

Before you can be considered for appointment with the NHS we need to be satisfied about your character and suitability.

The NHS aims to promote equality of opportunity and is committed to treating all applicants for positions fairly and on merit regardless of race, gender, marital status, religion or belief, disability, sexual orientation and age. The NHS undertakes not to discriminate unfairly against applicants on the basis of a criminal conviction or other information declared.

If you are applying for a post involving access to persons in receipt of health services, your offer of employment may be subject to a satisfactory disclosure from the Criminal Records Bureau. Failure to reveal information relating to any convictions could lead to withdrawal of an offer of employment.

Anyone applying for a position which involves a regulated activity and certain controlled activity from 12 October 2009 will require an enhanced Criminal Records Bureau check and that disclosure will, where appropriate to the role, include information against the Independent Safeguarding Authority barred lists for working with children or working with adults or both.

Are you currently bound over, or do you have any unspent convictions issued by a Court or Court Martial in the UK or any other country?
☐   Yes   ☐   No
If yes, please supply details below:

Rehabilitation of Offenders Act 1974 (Exceptions) Order 1975

To protect certain vulnerable groups within society, there are a number of posts within the NHS that are exempt from the provisions of the Rehabilitation of Offenders Act 1974. As the post you have applied for falls within this category, it will be exempt from the provisions of the Rehabilitation of Offenders Act by virtue of the Rehabilitation of Offenders Act 1974 (Exceptions) Order 1975.

Applicants for such posts are not entitled to withhold any information about convictions or other relevant criminal record information which for other purposes are 'spent' under the provisions of the Act. If you are successful with this application, any failure to disclose such information could result in dismissal or disciplinary action. Any information provided will be confidential and will be considered only in relation to posts to which the Order applies.

From 12 October 2009 under the terms of the Safeguarding Vulnerable Groups Act (2006), all positions involving regulated and certain controlled activity with children and vulnerable adults and which are carried out frequently, intensively or overnight will require an enhanced Disclosure and Barring Service (DBS formally Criminal Records Bureau) check. Where appropriate to the role, the DBS disclosure will include information against the Independent Safeguarding Authority barred lists for working with children and/or vulnerable adults.

Are you currently bound over or have you ever been convicted of any offence by a Court or Court-Martial in the United Kingdom or in any other country?
☐   Yes   ☐   No
If YES, please include details of the order binding you over and/or the nature of the offence, the penalty, sentence or order of the Court, and the date and place of the Court hearing. Please note: you do not need to tell us about parking offences.
Has your name ever appeared on the Protection of Children's List or have you ever been referred to the Independent Safeguarding Authority (ISA) for consideration of barring against the Children's List?
☐   Yes   ☐   No
Has your name ever appeared on the Protection of Vulnerable Adults List or have you ever been referred to the Independent Safeguarding Authority (ISA) for consideration of barring against the Vulnerable Adults List?
☐   Yes   ☐   No

Relationships

If you are related to a director, or have a relationship with a director or employee of an appointing organisation, please state the relationship.
The organisation needs to ensure there is no favouritism or bias in their appointments.

* DECLARATION The information from here on will go to the interviewers.

The information in this form is true and complete. I agree that any deliberate omission, falsification or misrepresentation in the application form will be grounds for rejecting this application or subsequent dismissal if employed by the organisation. Where applicable, I consent that the organisation can seek clarification regarding professional registration details.

(Continued)

Figure 8.3 (Continued)

I agree to the above declaration		
Signature		
Name	Full name	Date

Where did you see this vacancy advertised?			
☐ NHS Website	☐ Local Newspaper	☐ Doctor	☐ Nursing Standard
☐ Search Engine	☐ British Medical Journal	☐ Therapy Weekly	☐ Other Professional Journal
☐ Other Website	☐ Health Service Journal	☐ Nursing Times	☐ Jobcentre Plus
☐ National Newspaper	☐ Hospital Doctor	☐ GP	☐ Radio
			☐ Other

APPLICATION FOR EMPLOYMENT

Details entered in this part of the form will be held in the HR department of the recruiting organisation and will be made available to the short-listing panel.

Job Reference Number	Important to complete	Online reference number	This may be different from the job reference number
Job Title	Full job title		
Department	Name of department if known		

Education and Professional Qualifications may be required in chronological date order (newest to oldest)

Include in this section all the relevant qualifications. Please also indicate subjects currently being studied. All qualifications disclosed will be subject to a satisfactory check.			
Subject/Qualification	Place of Study	Grade/result	Year
Check the correct title of your University degree e.g. BSc Hons (RN Child)	University name	Pending, if not yet awarded	Month and year of qualification

Include in this section any relevant training courses that you have attended or details of courses that you are currently undertaking.			
Course Title	Training Provider	Duration	Date Completed
Include training that has been undertaken as part of your clinical placements, e.g. emergency CPR, cannulation, Acute Illness Management (AIM) training	Provide the relevant details in this and other sections.		

Membership of Professional Bodies

Include in this section any relevant professional registrations or memberships. If you are registered then please enter the relevant details below; this information will be subject to a satisfactory check. Indicate the information that is relevant to you at the time of application.

* Please indicate your Professional Registration status if relevant to this post:	
☐ I do not have the relevant UK professional registration status	☐ UK professional registration required but not yet applied for
☐ I have current UK professional registration	☐ I am a student
☐ UK professional registration required and applied for	☐ Not required for this post

If professional registration is not required then go to **Employment History**.

If you are registered then please enter the relevant details below:			
Professional Body	Membership or Registration type	Membership/ Registration PIN	Expiry/Renewal Date
Nursing and Midwifery Council	**Registered Nurse-Children**	**PENDING**	

If you are applying for a post that requires professional registration you are required to provide the following information. It is always best to answer honestly.

Are you currently the subject of a fitness to practise investigation or proceedings by an Education body or Regulatory body in the UK or in any other country?	☐ Yes ☐ No
Have you been removed from the register or have conditions been made on your registration by a fitness to practise committee or the licensing or regulatory body in the UK or in any other country?	☐ Yes ☐ No

If applicable, please provide details of any conditions/restrictions you may have.

Employment History

Please record below the details of your current or most recent employer

Employer Name	Just like the rest of the form, provide accurate details.		
	Do not answer this as your university as they do not employ you.		
Address			
Type of Business		Telephone	
Job Title			
Start Date		End Date	
Start of continuous NHS service			

Figure 8.3   (Continued)

Grade		Salary	
Reporting to (job title)		Notice Period	
Reason for leaving (if applicable)			
If you don't think that this information would be relevant then simply enter N/A.			
Description of your duties and responsibilities			
Get some value out of this experience. It may be unrelated to nursing but you will still be able to emphasise the development of transferable skills e.g. communication and interpersonal skills. Limit what you write; it's important to be concise.			

Previous Employment

Please record below the details of your most recent previous employment. If required, please provide additional information regarding your employment history within the **Supporting Information** section.

Previous Employer 1

Employer Name			
Address			
Job Title		Grade	
From Date		To Date	
Reason for Leaving			
See previous			
Description of your duties and responsibilities			
See previous			

Please add additional employers/information on a separate sheet.

If you have any gaps within your employment history, please state below.

Supporting Information: 1,500 words only

In this section please give your reasons for applying for this post and additional information which shows how you match the job description and person specification for the job (you will have been sent this document with the application form). Please include relevant skills; knowledge, experience, voluntary activities and training. If relevant to the post for which you are applying you should include details about research experience, publications or poster presentation, clinical care (knowledge and skills) and clinical audit.

Supporting Information (please continue on additional sheets if necessary).

This is the crucial section of the application. What you write here will be judged on a points scale and will determine whether you will be offered an interview.

Although how to approach your supporting statement is covered extensively within this chapter, it is worth reiterating how to approach this section of the application.

The key word to remember for this section is 'Evidence', this is what the interviewer will be looking for. Your evidence comes from your experience and needs to be communicated concisely. Within the NHS application form, you have 1,500 words, which amounts to roughly two pages of a Word document. You may not write this much and it is important to find a balance between depth and readability. Whoever is making a judgement on your suitability will be reading lots of these statements, so make it easy for them.

1. Break your statement down into shorter, readable sections.
2. State clearly your commitment to the profession and role being applied for. Demonstrate your knowledge of the Trust/company/ward/department/unit.
3. Follow the headings used in the person specification – address these individually if the person specification allows it; if not, provide summary statements covering a number of points. These need to be based in your experience.
4. Use the headings and points in the person specification to structure your statement into a series of short, focused statements.
5. Try to avoid, 'I feel, I believe' statements that reflect your opinion rather than fact. E.g. If you have good communication skills, what have you done that demonstrated this, and who would support it (Patients, Mentors, members of the multidisciplinary team)?
6. Conclude by re-stating your commitment to the profession, the Trust/employer and the role.

Hopefully, by approaching your statement in a clear and structured way will help you to demonstrate that you have the capability for the role. Always keep the person reading your form in mind. The easier it is to read, the greater your chances of being successful.

Additional Personal Information

Preferred Employment Type	☐ Full Time ☐ Part Time ☐ Job Share ☐ Secondment ☐ Flexible Hours
If applicable to the post, do you hold a certificate to support your responsibilities under IR (ME)R 2000?	☐ Yes ☐ No

References

Please state the names and contact details of the people who have agreed to supply references covering a minimum of 3 years employment/training/Education. If you are or have been employed, these should include your two most recent employers, your line manager or someone in a position of responsibility who can comment on your work experience, competence, personal qualities and suitability for the post. If you are a student please provide contact details of a teacher at your school, college or university. If you have not been in employment for a considerable amount of time but have had previous employment, then you should seek one reference from your last known employer and a personal reference from a person of some standing within your community i.e. doctor, solicitor, MP. Where it is not possible to obtain any employer reference at all then please obtain two personal references. Where no personal reference can be obtained then references should be sought from personal acquaintances not related to or involved in any financial arrangement with you. If you have undergone training to return to work, then the academic institution should be contacted. Personal references such as friends and relatives are not acceptable unless stated previously.

(Continued)

Figure 8.3 (Continued)

Please note, all reference requests will be sought through your line manager or other relevant department manager and your employment history will be verified through the organisation's Human Resources department or other relevant recruitment function. Please ensure that you provide full contact details. Referees may be contacted prior to interview.

Referee 1: Your current academic Personal Tutor

*Surname/Family name		First Name	
Title			
Job Title			
*Address			
*Post Code/Zip Code		*Country	
Telephone		Fax	
Email			
* Relationship		*Can the referee be contacted prior to interview?	☐ Yes ☐ No

Referee 2: Senior nursing practitioner (e.g. sign off mentor)

*Surname/Family name		First Name	
Title			
Job Title			
*Address			
*Post Code/ Zip Code		*Country	
Telephone		Fax	
Email			
* Relationship		* Can the referee be contacted prior to interview?	☐ Yes ☐ No

If you have applied to us within the last 3 months, are you happy for us to use the references from your earlier application?	☐ Yes ☐ No

Figure 8.3 Example application form

Preparing for and taking part in the interview process

On successful completion of your application you have been invited for interview. The following section provides information on the interview process and helps you to prepare for the process.

Values based recruitment (VBR)

It is worth noting at this point that in recent years the NHS and other organisations have been reviewing their recruitment practices in light of recent, critical reports into the standards of nursing and social care. A key report was the Francis Report (2013). In response to this and other reports the NHS has been developing, refining and implementing a 'values based recruitment approach'. Health Education England outlined the VBR approach as having the following characteristics:

* *Definition*: values based recruitment is an approach that attracts and selects students, trainees or employees on the basis that their individual values and behaviours align with the values of the NHS Constitution.
* *Purpose*: the purpose of values based recruitment is to ensure that the future and current NHS workforce is selected against the values of the NHS Constitution so that we have a workforce not only with the right skills, but with the right values to support effective team working in delivering excellent patient care and experience.
* *Delivery*: values based recruitment can be delivered in a number of ways: through pre-screening assessments, to values based interviewing techniques and role play, to scenarios and assessment centre approaches.

NHS employers: values-based recruitment interviews

Within your supporting statement be prepared to communicate how you have demonstrated these values within your clinical experience. For instance, one criterion within a person specification may be, 'Demonstrates an awareness of patient dignity and respect'. Providing specific evidence to show how you meet this criterion will have to include an expression of values. Perhaps you worked with a patient that was particularly distressed, or maybe you took time to speak to the family to prepare them for bad news? These would be appropriate examples to use to illustrate that you have the values. Don't be afraid to express these, but, if you are using a specific instance, please don't provide any personal details and don't forget to use STAR/CAR.

Choosing with care

Following the Warner report (1992) organisations with caring responsibilities have to ensure that they are employing the 'right' sort of people; this will involve you having an enhanced DBS check (www.gov.uk/disclosure-barring-service-check/overview).

Employers will also need to ensure you are who you say you are when you attend for interview. You will therefore be required to bring some form of photo ID, e.g. passport and/or driving licence, plus two documents that contain your name and current address.

The diagram in Figure 8.4 will help you to understand the stages of the recruitment process.

Preparing for the interview

An interview is essentially a performance, and like all performances, success depends on careful preparation and practice 'Fail to prepare, prepare to fail'.

Like Nusrat you may be at the stage where you do not really know what to expect from an interview. Support will be available for you at your university – the best place to start is to access resources from your Careers and Employability Service. Services that are available will include a talk with a careers advisor, access to a range of online resources, workshops and guides on the interview process.

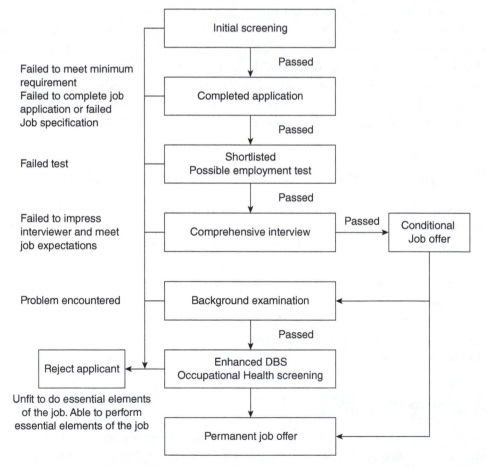

Figure 8.4 The selection process

The format of the selection process may not be the same for all the jobs that you apply for. If you have reached the short list there may be the following process:

Assessment centres can be used as a part of the recruitment process to reduce the numbers of candidates to be interviewed. Tests carried out at the centre may include:

- numeracy: medication calculations with or without a calculator;
- literacy: including the use of case studies or written scenarios;
- practical clinical skills assessment: to assess your ability in fundamental and core clinical skills;
- psychometric testing: to assess your values and attitudes;
- interviews – these could be either individual or group or both;
- role play – maybe with a member of the public or service user to assess your communication skills;
- presentations – normally timed, topic may be known beforehand or given on the day;
- group discussion – topic may be known or unknown.

To ensure fairness and equity, many interview panels use a point based system to score the quality and detail of your response to each question. They will then add up the scores for each applicant and award the job to the person with the most points, they will also have an expectation of the answers they are expecting to receive. Example of a scoring system:

Instructions for scoring interview: mark is 0–5

P = required prompting

0 = no answer/incorrect answer or information

1 = unsatisfactory answered very briefly or with much prompting

2 = adequate brief answer with no elaboration/no evidence/answered as a student

3 = fair answer with some explanations/some evidence of staff nurse role

4 = good answer with application of examples from experience/evidence of staff nurse role

5 = excellent answer showing insight, forward planning, explicit knowledge of role of the staff nurse – includes most of the cues from the answer column.

Getting there and what to wear

Getting there: Ensure you leave in plenty of time, it is better to be early and wait than to keep your interviewers waiting.

What to wear: Many students have asked this question, so it is an important one to consider. You want to appear professional and therefore you might want to choose your outfit carefully.

In preparation for a forthcoming interview Nusrat has been thinking about what to wear.

Activity 8.3   Decision making

List four Dos and Don'ts of what you would wear for an interview.

You could refer to the dress code policy of your local trust.

There is an outline answer to this activity at the end of the chapter.

The main point from this activity is that you are making an impression and you want to make a good one! First impressions count.

Researching possible interview questions

You might start to prepare for your interview by considering the questions that you are likely to be asked. Two of the most common questions are:

1   Tell me about yourself.

This is one of the most commonly used interview questions. The interviewer asks this to get a rounded sense of you as a person, and how you might fit within the team and organisation. The question seems informal, but don't drop your guard and ramble. Your interviewer is not looking for a 10-minute dissertation here. Instead, offer a focussed sentence or two that sets the stage for further discussion and, highlights your key skills, attitudes and personal objectives. This is an opportunity to show how you meet some of the Trust values. You also need to consider how you can use STAR/CAR to structure your answer.

DO

- mention impressive achievements early on;
- include enough information to give a rounded sense of you as a person; talk about you personally as well as professionally;
- give them 'your synopsis about you' answer, specifically your unique selling proposition, i.e. what makes you unique and suitable for the role.

DON'T

- ramble; keep things to a brief couple of minutes;
- assume the interviewer knows your background from your CV, they may have never read it.

2   Why did you apply for this job?

One of the most predictable questions. You need to demonstrate your knowledge of the employer (by reading employer brochures/annual reports/website/industry press) and link that knowledge in to a positive reason why you chose to apply. This is also an opportunity for you to positively highlight how you could contribute to the organisation and why this specific role fits the bill. Show enthusiasm for the role; the interviewer will want to know precisely why you selected them.

DO

- be positive, discuss your ambitions and values and explain why you think they are a good match to the role;
- have a specific reason as to why you are enthusiastic about what the organisation does;
- if possible, talk about any first-hand experience you've had, e.g. discussing the role with someone already performing it.

DON'T

- be negative, ensure that you have prepared a list of your ambitions and why this role meets them or can help you reach them;
- be complacent; even if you have a sufficient skill set a positive attitude is just as important;
- lie about wanting the role; if you don't genuinely believe the role fits you shouldn't be applying.

Scenario based questions:

While undertaking your nursing assessment you notice bruising on the patient. What would your actions be?

Structure your answer using **CAR**.

C – I had a similar situation on a surgical ward at the end of my final Year 2 placement.

A – As a student nurse, I asked the patient how they acquired the bruising, assessed their mobility using the appropriate assessment tool, ensured the extent of the bruising was clearly recorded on the appropriate documentation, e.g. body chart, and escalated my concerns to the safeguarding team. As a staff nurse I would do all of the afore-mentioned actions, ensuring that the appropriate Trust procedures and policies were followed and implemented.

R – The patient was assessed as being prone to falls and the appropriate interventions were put in place during their period of hospitalisation and when they were discharged home.

Further interview questions

If the organisation where you are being interviewed has adopted a Values Based Recruitment approach (see above), then you might find the style a little different from the normal 'competency' based interview. Here you will have a lead question, followed up with a number of probing questions, designed to get to the heart of what motivates and influences your actions and behaviour. Here are some examples to give you a flavour:

- Can you give an example of where you've spoken up because you had concerns?
  - o How did it feel to you?
  - o What were the outcomes?
  - o If it was a successful intervention – why do you think it was successful?
  - o If it was not a successful intervention – why do you think this was the case? What did you learn from this episode about yourself?

- Tell me about a time when you have 'gone the extra mile' within your clinical experience.
  - o What did you do?
  - o Why did you do that?
  - o What was the outcome?

- Can you give an example of how you developed compassion for a person you were caring for?
  - o Reflecting on the experience what did you learn?
  - o How did you use the experience to develop your practice further?

As you can see, the questioning style goes to a much greater depth and is aimed at moving you away from rehearsed responses. CAR still works well in this situation. You will be required to provide an example from your experience, but as you can see from the probing questions, you will be required to reflect on the situation to a much greater degree than is the case when answering a pure competency question.

Answering the questions

Take time to consider what has been asked. You can ask them to repeat the question. Don't waffle but do expand on your answer. You might use examples from your knowledge and experience.

Taking part in a mock interview

Your university may have a system where you can participate in a mock interview. This process can really help by simulating the experience and providing you with some feedback on your performance. It can also help you to reflect on your performance and think about what you did well and areas for improvement.

What evidence shall I bring?

Many students ask this question before attending an interview. How do you decide whether to take your portfolio to the interview? As part of your undergraduate programme you will have most likely developed a vast amount of evidence that demonstrates the development of your knowledge, skills and values throughout your programme of study. However, it may not be practical to take all this evidence with you for the interview. Interviewers may have limited time, so better to bring a small amount of evidence that clearly demonstrates your suitability for the post, in terms of the knowledge, skills and values. This also demonstrates that you have taken the time to think about what is most relevant. It is also a good idea to refer to this evidence when you are answering the questions, rather than a large portfolio that people may just flick through and not remember.

Employers may have expectations of what they are looking for at interview.

Employers' expectations

Activity 8.4   Critical thinking

Employers report that at interview they can identify the way in which newly registered nurses have met or not met their expectations. For example, your interviewers are looking for you to demonstrate baseline competencies, knowledge, skills and values. These include: communication, literacy, numeracy, medicines management, clinical skills, values, clinical judgement.

Make a list of what you think employer's expectations might be.

Now consider how you can ensure that you meet employer expectations. For example, consider how you would demonstrate motivation for the job.

There is an outline answer to this activity at the end of the chapter.

Examples of newly registered nurses not meeting employer's expectations include:

- poor motivation and lack of enthusiasm for the job;
- poor appearance: scruffiness and inappropriate dress;
- lack of respect for co-workers and patients;
- lack of confidence in the ability to do the job;
- poor clinical knowledge and skills: particularly relating to medication;
- poor reporting skills: written and verbal;
- poor understanding of role and what was expected from them;
- poor documentation, particularly the language used;

- overconfidence and rash decision making;
- not working as a team;
- high sickness and absence;
- lack of empathy and care.

You might want to reflect on these and consider ways of addressing them in your preparation for interview. For example, if you have a high sickness and absence you might explain the reason for this in your interview.

Managing nerves and stress

You may find the interview process itself stressful and nerve-wracking. For ways to manage nerves and stress, see Chapter 4.

Reflecting on the interview process

Whether or not you are successful at interview it is important to reflect on the process and identify what you did well and areas for development. Refer to the Chapter 3 on reflection for strategies to do this. In addition to self-assessment and reflection, ask for feedback from the interviewer.

Preparing to start your career

Congratulations you have been successful in starting your nursing career! Now

1. consider the academic knowledge, professional skills, personal attitude and characteristics that you might need to develop for your new post; consider e.g. for Personal Attitude: team working style, breaking bad news, communication style;

2. undertake a SWOT/SNOB analysis around these areas;

3. develop PDPs to address your areas for development during your preceptorship period (see Chapter 6);

4. identify five patients within the clinical area: what are the main diseases/conditions they have? Consider the related anatomy and physiology, treatment options, nursing care required;

5. find out the ten most common drugs used in this clinical area; consider common dose, effects, side effects, and contraindications;

6. consider the Trust policies and procedures; lone working, infection control, medicine policy;

7. consider how you can use the information from your preceptorship period towards your NMC revalidation in 3 years' time.

Chapter summary

This chapter has examined all aspects of the process of applying for your first post. Key elements of the application process have been discussed including analysis of job descriptions and person specifications. Strategies have been identified for completing the application form and the personal statement. Taking part in the interview or assessment process itself has been discussed and ideas for further development once you have secured the post explored.

Activities: brief outline answers

Activity 8.1 Critical thinking (page 159)

One statement on a recent job description for a band 5 Registered Children's Nurse was:

Promote the concept of family centred care – you might consider your recent assignment of family centred case as evidence. You have also been assessed as competent to deliver child and family-centred care by your recent mentor on your clinical placement.

Activity 8.2 Decision making (page 161)

Skills/Abilities	Evidence/Examples
Ability to plan and prioritise care for patients.	I have been assessed as competent in assessing, planning and prioritising care in all my practice placements. My mentor commented that I had excellent skills in this area. I have managed a group of 6 patients on my recent placement. I have experience of using care plans including integrated case pathways for example.

Table 8.2 Evidence from self-assessment

Activity 8.3 Decision making (page 180)

DO dress to impress

DO wear something smart but comfortable

DON'T let your clothes be a distraction

DON'T wear something too tight or too revealing

Activity 8.4 Critical thinking (page 183)

- Expectations from employers at interview (Burke *et al.*, 2014):
  - excellent communication skills: written, verbal and non-verbal;
  - good basic core clinical skills;
  - good clinical judgement;
  - professional attitude: punctuality and reliability;

    o   ability to work in a team;

    o   awareness of own limitations and to know when to seek help;

- Willingness and enthusiasm to learn:
  o   excellent assessment and evaluation skills;
  o   commitment to doing a good job.

Further reading

Knight, P and Yorke, M (2004) *Learning, curriculum and employability in higher education.* London: Routledge Falmer, in Cole, D and Tibby, M (eds) (2013) *Defining and Developing Your Approach to Employability: A framework for higher education institutions.* York: Higher Education Academy. www.heacademy.ac.uk/knowledge-hub/defining-and-developing-your-approach-employability-framework-higher-education

This document is a framework for reflecting on and addressing employability in a systematic and holistic way.

The Equality Act 2010. www.legislation.gov.uk/ukpga/2010/15/contents

The Equality Act protects you from various forms of discrimination relating to disability, and also discrimination and harassment. Direct discrimination is when you are treated less favourably than another person because of your disability.

Royal College of Nursing (2016) *The RCN Reasonable Adjustments: The peer support service guide for members affected by disability in the workplace.* London: RCN. www.rcn.org.uk/professional-development/publications/pub-005756

This publication recognises that people with impairments are able to undertake employment and are an available resource. It offers guidance on how changes to workplace environments and attitudes can assist in ensuring that employees with impairments have a fair opportunity to work to the best of their abilities.

The RCN Dyslexia, Dyspraxia and Dyscalculia: A toolkit for nursing staff. www.rcn.org.uk/professional-development/publications/pub-003835

This guidance will support nursing staff with specific learning differences, their colleagues and their managers to realise their full potential and continue to make a valuable contribution to healthcare.

Warner, N (1992) *Choosing with Care: The Report of the Committee of Inquiry into the Selection, Development and Management of Staff in Children's Homes.* London: HMSO.

This report highlights the need to improve training around the selection of candidates to work with children.

Useful websites

The RCN Learning Zone can help you improve your numeracy skills.

www.rcn.org.uk/learningzone

The Graduate Careers Website, Prospects, provides guidance on preparing for assessment centres.

www.prospects.ac.uk/assessment_centres.htm

Accessing relevant online resources to start your nursing career

www.jobs.nhs.uk/

NHS Jobs is a dedicated online recruitment service for the NHS. Every NHS organisation within England and Wales advertises their job opportunities with NHS Jobs. In addition a number of organisations outside the NHS have chosen to advertise their health related vacancies on NHS Jobs too.

www.rcn.org.uk/professional-development/find-a-job

Whether you're applying for your first job, looking for career progression or moving to a more senior position as a healthcare professional, the RCN careers service has information and resources that can guide you to make decisions about your career.

www.nhsprofessionals.nhs.uk

NHSP currently have hundreds of flexible work opportunities for short and long-term positions across all specialities.

As the leader of flexible worker managed services to the NHS we have a significant number of positions available daily – you can view these Hot Jobs using the following links to NHS Jobs:

www.nursingnetuk.com/job

An information service for nurses website to cover all health sector jobs.

Country specific careers services:

England **https://nationalcareersservice.direct.gov.uk**

Wales **www.careerswales.com/en/**

Scotland **www.skillsdevelopmentscotland.co.uk**

Northern Ireland **www.nidirect.gov.uk/front**

These sites provide information, advice and guidance to help you make decisions on learning, training and work.

References

Akerjordet, K and Severinsson, E (2008) Emotionally intelligent nurse leadership: A literature review study. *Journal of Nursing Management, 16*: 565–77.

American Psychological Association (2016) The Road to Resilience: 10 ways to build resilience. www.apa.org/helpcenter/road-resilience.aspx

Bauer, WI and Dunn, RE (2003) Digital reflection: The electronic portfolio in music teacher education. *Journal of Music Teacher Education, 13*(1): 7–21.

Bandura, A (1997a) *Self-Efficacy: The Exercise of Control.* New York: WH Freeman.

Bandura, A (1977b) *Social Learning Theory.* London: Prentice-Hall.

Belbin, M (1981) *Management Teams.* London: Heinemann, www.belbin.com/about/belbin-team-roles/

Benner, P (1982) From novice to expert. *The American Journal of Nursing, 82*(3): 402–7.

Bloom, BS and Krathwohl, DR (1956) *Taxonomy of Educational Objectives: The Classification of Educational Goals, by a committee of college and university examiners. Handbook I: Cognitive Domain.* New York: Longmans, Green.

Bloom, BS, Krathwhol, DR and Masia, BB (1964) *Taxonomy of Educational Objectives: Volume II, The Affective Domain.* New York: David McKay.

Boronski, T and Hassan, N (2015) *Sociology of Education.* London: Sage.

Borton, T (1970) *Reach, Touch and Teach: Student concerns and process education.* New York: McGraw Hill.

Bourdieu, P and Passeron, J-C (2000) *Reproduction in Education, Society and Culture.* London: Sage.

Boychuk Duchscher, J (2007) *Professional role transition into acute-care by newly qualified graduated baccalaureate female registered nurses.* Unpublished PhD thesis. University of Alberta, Canada.

British Association for Counselling and Psychotherapy (2017) Stress Test. www.bbc.co.uk/news/health-24756311

Burke, L, Sayer, J, Morris-Thompson, T and Marks-Maran, D (2014) Recruiting competent newly qualified nurses in the London region: An exploratory study. *Nurse Education Today, 34*: 1283–9.

Burton, R and Ormrod, G (Eds) (2011) *Nursing: Transition to professional practice.* Oxford: Oxford University Press.

Butts, J and Rich, K (2014) *Philosophies and Theories for Advanced Nursing Practice* (2nd edn). Burlington, IN: Jones & Bartlett.

Carper, BA (1978) Fundamental patterns of knowing in nursing. *Advances in Nursing Science, 1*(1): 13–24.

Chan, ZCY (2014) Students' and experts' perspectives on three learning and teaching activities. *Nurse Education in Practice, 14*(5): 449–54.

Chapman, A (1995–2014) Johari Window Alan Chapman adaptation, review and code 1995–2014, based on Ingham and Luft's original Johari Window concept. www.businessballs.com/johariwindowmodel.htm

Chapman, L (2013) A 'roll-on, roll-off' preceptorship pathway for new registrants. *Nursing Management, 20*(2): 24–6.

Chen, G, Gully, S and Eden, D (2001) Validation of a new general self-efficacy scale. *Organizational Research Methods, 4*: 62–83. http://orm.sagepub.com/content/4/1/62.full.pdf+html

Chesser-Smyth, P (2013) How to build self-confidence. *Nursing Standard, 27*(52): 64.

Chick, N and Meleis, A (1986) Transitions: A nursing concern, in Chinn, P (ed) *Nursing Research Methodology: Issues and implementation.* Rockville, MD: Aspen.

Clark, T and Holmes, S (2007) Fit for practice? An exploration of the development of newly qualified nurses using focus groups. *International Journal of Nursing Studies, 44*: 1210–20.

Coffield, F, Moseley, D, Hall, E, and Ecclestone, K (2004) *Learning Styles and Pedagogy in Post-16 Learning: A systematic and critical review.* London: Learning and Skills Research Centre.

Coleman, D and Willis, DS (2015) Reflective writing: The student nurse's perspective on reflective writing and poetry writing. *Nurse Education Today, 35*(7): 906–11.

Covey, S (1989) *The 7 habits of highly effective people.* New York: Freepress.

Cowan, J (2010) Developing the ability for making evaluative judgements. *Teaching in Higher Education, 15*(3): 323–34. www.tandfonline.com/doi/abs/10.1080/13562510903560036

Coward, M (2011) Does the use of reflective models restrict critical thinking and therefore learning in nurse education? What have we done? *Nurse Education Today, 31*(8): 883–6.

Crooks, D, Brown, B, Black, M, O'Mara, I and Noesgaard, C (2005) Development of professional confidence by post diploma baccalaureate nursing students. *Nurse Education in Practice, 5*, 360–7.

Croughan, CE (2016) Student nurses' preparation and negotiation of transition to the registered nurse role. Are there any factors that influence or inhibit this successful negotiation and transition? A systematic review. *Unpublished MSc thesis, University of Salford.* http://usir.salford.ac.uk/38397/

Darvill, A (2013) A qualitative study into the experiences of newly qualified children's nurses during their transition into children's community nursing teams. Unpublished PhD thesis. *University of Salford.* http://usir.salford.ac.uk/38397/

Darvill, A, Fallon, D and Livesley, J (2014) A different world? The transition experiences of newly qualified children's nurses taking up first destination posts within children's community nursing teams. *Issues in Comprehensive Paediatric Nursing, 37*(1): 6–24.

Dave, RH (1970) Developing and writing behavioral objectives. www.businessballs.com/bloomstaxonomyoflearningdomains.htm

Davis, SE (1945) What are modern martyrs worth. *Peabody Journal of Education, 23*(2): 67–8.

Dearing Report (1997) *Higher Education in the Learning Society.* London: HMSO.

De Bono, E (2016) *Six Thinking Hats.* London: Penguin Life.

Department of Health (2004) *NHS Knowledge and Skills Framework (NHS KSF) and the Development Review Process.* London: Department of Health.

Department of Health (2010) *Preceptorship Framework for Newly Registered Nurses, Midwives and Allied Health Professionals.* London: Department of Health.

Dewey, J (1933) *How We Think.* Boston, MA: DC Heath.

Dohrenwend, A (2002) Serving up the feedback sandwich. *Family Practice Manager, 9*(10): 43–5.

Doran, GT (1981) There's a S.M.A.R.T. way to write management's goals and objectives. *Management Review, 70*(11): 35–6.

Driscoll, J (1994) Reflective practice for practise: A framework of structured reflection for clinical areas. *Senior Nurse, 14*(1): 47.

Duchscher, JEB (2009) Transition shock: The initial stage of role adaptation for newly graduated registered nurses. *Journal of Advanced Nursing, 65*(5): 1103–13.

Duffy, K (2013) Providing constructive feedback to students during mentoring. *Nursing Standard, 27*(31): 50–6.

Evans, J, Boxer, E, and Sanber, S (2008) The strengths and weaknesses of transitional support programs for newly registered nurses. *Australian Journal of Advanced Nursing, 25*(4): 16–22.

Fisher, J (2012) Fisher's process of personal change – revised 2012. *John Fisher's personal transition curve – the stages of personal change.* www.businessballs.com/personalchangeprocess.htm

Fleming, ND and Mills, C (1992) Not another inventory, rather a catalyst for reflection. *To Improve the Academy, 11*: 137–144.

Fosnot, C (2005) *Constructivism: Theory, perspectives and practice* (2nd edn). New York: Teachers College Press.

Francis, R (2013) *Report of the Mid Staffordshire NHS Foundation Trust Public Inquiry.* London: The Stationery Office.

Getselfhelp (2015) Self Help for Stress. www.getselfhelp.co.uk/stress.htmc

Gibbs, G (1988) *Learning by Doing: A guide to teaching and learning methods.* Oxford: Further Education Unit Oxford Polytechnic.

Goldblatt, PF (2006) How John Dewey's theories underpin art and art education. *Education and Culture, 22*(1): 17–34.

Grant, L and Kinman, G (2014) Emotional resilience in the helping professions and how it can be enhanced. *Health and Social Care Education, 3*(1): 23–34.

Harrow, AJ (1972) A taxonomy of the psychomotor domain: A guide for developing behavioural objectives. www.businessballs.com/bloomstaxonomyoflearningdomains.htm

Helms, MM and Nixon, J (2010) Exploring SWOT analysis – where are we now? A review of academic research from the last decade. *Journal of Strategy and Management, 3*(3): 215–251.

Hewitt, PL and Flett, GL (1991) Perfectionism in the self and social contexts: Conceptualization, assessment, and association with psychopathology. *Journal of Personality and Social Psychology, 60*: 456–70.

Honey, P and Mumford, A (1992) *The Manual of Learning Styles: Revised version.* Maidenhead, UK: Peter Honey.

Honey, P and Mumford, A (2000) *The Learning Styles Questionnaire 80-item Version.* Maidenhead, UK: Honey P Publications. http://resources.eln.io/honey-mumford-learner-types-1986-questionnaire-online

Humphrey, AS (2005) SWOT Analysis for Management Consulting. *SRI Alumni Association Newsletter,* December. www.sri.com/sites/default/files/brochures/dec-05.pdf

Johns, C (1995) Framing learning through reflection within Carper's fundamental ways of knowing in nursing. *Journal of Advanced Nursing, 22*(2): 226–34.

Kearns, H (2016) The Imposter Syndrome: Why successful people often feel like frauds. http://impostersyndrome.com.au/index.php/the-free-guide/

Kegan, R (1983) *The Evolving Self: Problem and process in human development.* Cambridge, MA: Harvard University Press.

Kellogg, R (2002) *Cognative Psychology* (2nd edn). London: Sage.

Kolb, D (1984) *Experiential Learning as the Science of Learning and Development.* Englewood Cliffs, NJ: Prentice Hall.

Kramer, M (1974) *Reality Shock: Why nurses leave nursing.* St Louis, MO: Mosby.

Krathwohl, DR and Anderson, LW (2010) Merlin C. Wittrock and the revision of Bloom's Taxonomy. *Educational Psychologist, 45*(1): 64–5. www.tandfonline.com/doi/full/10.1080/00461520903433562

Lave, J and Wenger, E (1991) *Situated Learning: Legitimate peripheral participation.* Cambridge: Cambridge University Press.

Leigh, JA, Williamson, T and Rutherford, J (2017) Stakeholder perspectives of an approach to healthcare leadership development through use of a multidimensional leadership development conceptual model. *International Journal of Practice-based Learning in Health and Social Care, 5*(1): 77–97.

Likert, R (1932) A technique for the measurement of attitudes. *Archives of Psychology, 140*: 1–55.

Luft, J (1969) *Of Human Interaction: The Johari Model.* Palo Alto, CA: Mayfield. www.businessballs.com/johariwindowmodel.htm

Mahony, DL, Burroughs, WJ and Lippman, LG (2002) Perceived attributes of health-promoting laughter: A cross-generational comparison. *Journal of Psychology, 136*: 171–81.

Major, DA (2010) Student nurses in transition: Generating an evidence base for final placement learning-facilitation best practice. MPhil Thesis. *University of Salford, Manchester, UK.*

Major, DA (2015) The effects of using transition-focused personal development plans on final year student nurses' personal qualities for learning. *University of Salford in-house research, Unpublished.* Manchester, UK: University of Salford.

Mandy, A and Tinley, P (2004) Burnout and occupational stress: Comparison between United Kingdom and Australian podiatrists. *Journal of American Podiatric Medical Association, 94*(3): 282–91.

Meleis, AI, Sawyer, LM, Im, EO, Hilfinger Messias, DK and Schumacher, K (2000) Experiencing transition: An emerging middle-range theory. *Advances in Nursing Science, 23*, 12–28.

Melling, S (2011) Transition: An exploration of student nurse experience in their first practice placement. *University of Nottingham.* http://eprints.nottingham.ac.uk/12157/

Mezirow, J (1991) *Transformative Dimensions of Adult Learning.* San Francisco, CA: Jossey-Bass.

Morley, M (2009) An evaluation of a SNP programme for newly qualified occupational therapists. *British Journal of Occupational Therapy, 72*(9): 384–92.

Morrell, N and Ridgway, V (2014) Are we preparing student nurses for their final placement? *British Journal of Nursing, 23*(10): 518–23.

Myers, I and Briggs, K (1962) The Myers-Briggs Type Indicator. *The Myers & Briggs Foundation.* www.myersbriggs.org/my-mbti-personality-type/mbti-basics/

Nash, R, Lemcke, P and Sacre, S (2009) Enhancing transition: An enhanced model of clinical placement for final year nursing students. *Nurse Education Today, 29*(1): 48–56.

National Health Service England (2016/05) *Leading Change, Adding Value: A framework for nursing midwifery and care staff.* www.England.nhs.uk.

National Health Executive (2015) More nurses off due to stress as NHS demand rises. www.nationalhealthexecutive.com/Workforce-and-Training/more-nurses-off-due-to-stress-as-nhs-demand-rises

National Health Service Leadership Academy (2013) NHS Healthcare Leadership Model. www.leadershipacademy.nhs.uk/resources/healthcare-leadership-model/

National Health Service Leadership Academy (2015) NHS Healthcare Leadership Model self-assessment tool. www.leadershipacademy.nhs.uk/resources/healthcare-leadership-model/supporting-tools-resources/healthcare-leadership-model-self-assessment-tool/

NHS Scotland (2010) *Effective Practitioner.* www.effectivepractitioner.nes.scot.nhs.uk/

Northouse, P (2015) *Leadership Theory and Practice* (7th edn). Thousand Oaks, CA: Sage.

Nursing and Midwifery Council (2006) Preceptorship guidelines. *NMC Circular 21/2006*. www.nmc.org.uk/globalassets/sitedocuments/circulars/2006circulars/nmc-circular-21_2006.pdf

Nursing and Midwifery Council (2010) *Standards for Pre-registration Nursing Education.* London: NMC.

Nursing and Midwifery Council (2014) *Standards for Competence for Registered Nurses.* London: NMC.

Nursing and Midwifery Council (2015) *The Code. Professional standards of practice and behaviour for nurses and midwives.* London: NMC.

Ong, G-L (2013) Using final placements to prepare student nurses. *Nursing Times, 109*(3): 12–14.

Pavlov, I (1960) *Conditioned Reflexes: An investigation of the physiological activity of the cerebral cortex.* New York: Dover Books.

Pepper, JR, Jaggar, SI, Mason, MJ, Finney, SJ and Dusmet, M (2012) Schwartz rounds: Reviving compassion in modern healthcare. *Journal of the Royal Society of Medicine, 105*(3): 94–5.

Philips, C, Estermann, A and Kenny, A (2015) The theory of organisational socialisation and its potential for improving transition experiences for new graduate nurses. *Nurse Education Today, 35*: 118–24.

Pitt, V, Powis, D, Levett-Jones, T and Hunter, S (2014) The influence of personal qualities on performance and progression in a pre-registration nursing programme. *Nurse Education Today, 34*(5): 866–71.

Quality Assurance Agency for Higher Education (2007) Using focused learner questions in personal development planning to support effective learning.www.qaa.ac.uk/en/Publications/Documents/Effective-Learning-Framework-Using-focused-learner-questions-in-personal-development-planning-to-support-effective-learning.pdf

Quality Assurance Agency (2008) *Framework for Higher Education Qualifications in England, Wales and Northern Ireland.* Gloucester, UK: QAA. www.qaa.ac.uk

Roach, MS (2002) *Caring, the Human Mode of Being: A blueprint for the health professions* (2nd edn). Ottawa, Canada: CHA Press.

Robinson, S and Griffiths, P (2008) *Scoping Review: Moving to an all-graduate nursing profession: Assessing potential effects on workforce profile and quality of care.* London: National Nursing Research Unit, King's College.

Rodgers, C (2002) Defining reflection: Another look at John Dewey and reflective thinking. *Teachers College Record, 104*(4): 842–66.

Royal College of Nursing (2002) Clinical supervision in the workplace. www.rcn.org.uk/-/media/royal-college-of-nursing/.../2003/pub-001549.pdf

Royal College of Nursing (2005) *NHS Knowledge and Skills Framework Outlines for Nursing Posts.* London: Royal College of Nursing.

Royal College of Nursing (2014) Defining nursing. www.rcn.org.uk/professional-development/publications/pub-004768

Royal College of Nursing (n.d.) Leadership programme. www.rcn.org.uk/professional-development/professional-services/leadership-programmes

Schön, DA (1983) *The Reflective Practitioner: How professionals think in action* (Vol 5126). New York: Basic books.

Schön, D (1987) *Educating the Reflective Practitioner.* Thousand Oaks, CA: Jossey-Bass.

Schutte, NS, Malouff, JM and Bhullar, N (2009) The assessing emotions scale, in Stough, C, Saklofske D and Parker, J (eds) *Assessing Emotional Intelligence: Theory, research and applications.* New York: Springer. www.researchgate.net/publication/216626162_The_Assessing_Emotions_Scale

Simpson, EJ (1972) The classification of educational objectives in the Psychomotor domain. www.businessballs.com/bloomstaxonomyoflearningdomains.htm

Skinner, B (1969) *Contingencies of Reinforcement: A theoretical analysis.* New York: Appleton-Century-Crofts.

Spouse, J (1998) Learning to nurse through legitimate peripheral participation. *Nurse Education Today, 18*(5): 345–51.

Standing, M (2017) *Clinical Judgement and Decision Making in Nursing* (3rd edn). London: Sage.

Steel, P (2007) The nature of procrastination: A meta-analytic and theoretical review of quintessential self-regulatory failure. *Psychological Bulletin, 133*(1): 65–94.

Strauss, E, Ovnat, C, Gonen, A, Lev-Ari, L and Mizrahi, A (2015) Do orientation programs help new graduates? *Nurse Education Today, 36*: 422–26.

Sykes, AE (2012) *Making the Most of Feedback: One step towards getting the most marks you can.* Manchester, UK: University of Salford. www.careers.salford.ac.uk/cms/resources/uploads/files/Making%20the%20Most%20of%20Feedback%20BINDER.pdf

van Gennep, A (1960) *The Rites of Passage.* London: Routledge.

van de Ridder, JM, Stokking, KM, McGaghie, WC and ten Cate, OTJ (2008) What is feedback in clinical education? *Medical Education, 42*: 189–97.

Warburton, T, Houghton, T and Barry, D (2016) Facilitation of learning: Part 1. *Nursing Standard, 30*(32): 40–7.

Warner, N (1992) Choosing with Care. *The Report of the Committee of Inquiry into the Selection, Development and Management of Staff in Children's Homes.* London: HMSO.

Weir-Hughes, D (2016) Editorial: Valuing the knowledge of nursing: Naming it and making it visible. *Journal of Clinical Nursing,* 25(13–14): 1787–8.

Weston, MJ (2010) Strategies for enhancing autonomy and control over nursing practice. *The Online Journal of Issues in Nursing, 15*(1): Manuscript 2.

Whitehead, B, Owen, P, Holmes, D, Beddingham, E, Simmons, M, Henshaw, L, Barton, M and Walker, C (2013) Supporting newly qualified nurses in the UK: A systematic literature review. *Nurse Education Today, 33*: 370–7.

Widdowson, M (2014) Avoidance, vicious cycles, and experiential disconfirmation of script: Two new theoretical concepts and one mechanism of change in the psychotherapy of depression and anxiety. *Transactional Analysis Journal, 44*(3): 194–207.

Willis Commission (2012) Shape of Caring: A review of the future education and training of registered nurses and care assistants. www.hee.nhs.uk/sites/default/files/documents/2348-Shape-of-caring-review-FINAL.pdf

World Health Organization (1946) Constitution of the World Health Organization as adopted by the International Health Conference, New York, 19–22 June 1946; signed on 22 July 1946 by the representatives of 61 States (Official Records of the World Health Organization, no. 2, p100) and entered into force on 7 April 1948. In Grad, Frank P (2002). The preamble of the constitution of the World Health Organization. Bulletin of the World Health Organization, *80*(12): 982.

World Health Organization (1982) Medium Term Programme. Geneva: WHO.

Yura, H and Walsh, MB (1973) *The Nursing Process: Assessing, planning, implementing, evaluating* (2nd edn). New York: Appleton-Century-Crofts.

Zamanzadeh, V, Jasemi, V, Valizadeh, L, Keogh, B and Taleghani, B (2015) Lack of preparation: Iranian nurses' experiences during transition from college to clinical practice. *Journal of Professional Nurse, 31*: 365–73.

Index